Practical
NURSING
Calculations

Practical
NURSING
Calculations

GETTING THE DOSE RIGHT

Valda Hext and Lidia Mayner

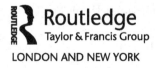

Routledge
Taylor & Francis Group

LONDON AND NEW YORK

To present and future nursing students.
Experience has shown that making nursing calculations is not only
simpler than you imagine, but also essential to the safe care of your
clients.

First published 2003 by Allen & Unwin

Published 2020 by Routledge
2 Park Square, Milton Park, Abingdon, Oxon OX14 4RN
605 Third Avenue, New York, NY 10017

Routledge is an imprint of the Taylor & Francis Group, an informa business

National Library of Australia
Cataloguing-in-Publication entry:

Hext, Valda.
    Practical nursing calculations: getting the dose right.

    Bibliography.
    ISBN 1 86508 874 9.

    1. Nursing – Mathematics. 2. Pharmaceutical arithmetic.
    I. Title

610.73

Set in 10/12 pt Simoncini Garamond by Midland Typesetters Pty Ltd, Maryborough, Victoria

ISBN-13: 9781865088747 (pbk)

CONTENTS

PREFACE

With calculators so readily available, many students assume that there is no need to be competent in basic mathematical skills. However, research carried out into the mathematical skills and conceptual ability of students enrolled in undergraduate nursing degrees in tertiary institutions in Victoria and South Australia indicates deficiencies which often hinder performance and cause considerable stress to the students throughout the course. This research also suggested that many students were unable to use a calculator with competence.

While calculators are a great asset, one also needs to take into account:

- they are not always available
- a basic understanding of arithmetic is often necessary to use a calculator, and
- it is important to know whether the answer *looks* correct because it is so easy to make mistakes when pushing buttons.

With the above information in mind, this book has been developed to assist students to gain competencies in basic mathematical skills and problem-solving techniques which require applied or conceptual mathematics. While many formulae have been used to calculate problems, it is important to remember that a logical or common sense approach is also useful.

This book has been prepared in six modules, one for each semester of the undergraduate three-year nursing degree course. It is set out in such a way that students have the opportunity to complete ten exercises each semester. The purpose of this is to develop new skills slowly, to foster understanding of what is being undertaken and to further enhance comprehension by repetition.

A large part of this book is based on clinical presentations of actual case studies by year two and three students while experiencing clinical placements.

Unless the learning institution where the student is studying permits the use of calculators, it is expected that the computations will be performed by the student by hand. The use of a calculator to *check* answers on completion of work is encouraged.

This workbook begins with a fairly comprehensive test of the mathematical skills needed to compute nursing calculations used during the three-year undergraduate degree program for nursing students. The purpose of the actual test is for students to identify any areas of weakness in mathematics and/or within the metric system, so that greater attention can be given to these areas.

Answers are available so that students can assess their progress. Where a greater understanding of a concept is necessary, the targeted area can be found in the index or on the Practical Nursing Calculations website at:

www.routledge.com/9781865088747

Also, several quizzes are available on this website for students to assess their knowledge and understanding of the covered topics, followed by extra practice should this be required.

Concepts are introduced gradually to allow students to grasp a new idea, following significant repetition of the previous topic. The complexity of the computations increases throughout the book until the point is reached where a student should be able to problem solve and compute calculations for any situation that could arise.

The nursing scenarios that are presented throughout the book are factual case studies presented by students while on their various clinical placements. It is acknowledged that some of the scenarios may contain medication orders which are questionable; these orders have been deliberately included to encourage students to develop a critical approach to the care that they give to the clients, particularly in relation to medication administration.

It is anticipated that students will enjoy working through the scenarios, and hopefully will not only understand the computations required, but will also begin to link the medications prescribed to the disease process.

ACKNOWLEDGEMENTS

Sincere thanks are expressed to the students from St Alban's Campus, Victoria University of Technology, and to students from Flinders University and the University of South Australia who contributed the scenarios used in modules three to six. It is recognised that a considerable amount of research into the medications used—their effects, both desirable and undesirable, interactions and correct dosages—has been contributed by the students.

In particular, Debbie Robinson, Rebecca Freer, Bronwen Donges, Andrea Byrne, Maria Blondell, Sarah Rosetti, Rebecca Hall, Gary Pentland and Katie Bowley.

To Judith Manning for her advice, ideas and time; to Jean-Pierre Calabretto who spent many hours considering the paediatric section and advising where necessary; to Jill Peisach for her assistance in high dependency and emergency nursing—thank you.

The authors would like to thank Flinders Medical Centre for permission to use their fluid balance and observation charts.

1

Basic Skills

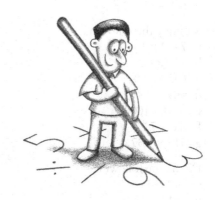

Objectives

After completing the given calculations, it is expected that you should be able to:

1 calculate basic mathematical problems such as
   - addition
   - subtraction
   - multiplication
   - division

2 apply the above skills to decimal calculations

3 add, subtract, multiply and divide fractions

4 identify the basic units of measurement in the metric system

5 understand the concept of ratios

INTRODUCTORY ASSESSMENT

1   Add the following
   a   93 + 147 + 6 + 8253
   b   11 + 27 + 113 + 2954
   c   64.8 + 724.36 + 27
   d   36 + 0.74 + 925

2   Subtract the following
   a   628 – 361
   b   7492 – 396
   c   1006.4 – 329.8
   d   629 – 46.8

3   Multiply the following
   a   7432 × 18
   b   231 × 62
   c   6428 × 10
   d   469 × 100
   e   63.8 × 1000
   f   8.6 × 7.2
   g   318 × 0.37

4   Divide the following
   a   612 ÷ 3
   b   9612 ÷ 12
   c   783.9 ÷ 100
   d   643 ÷ 1000
   e   468 ÷ 10
   f   132 ÷ 2.2
   g   1651 ÷ 2.54

5   Simplify the following fractions
   a $\dfrac{60}{90}$

   b $\dfrac{100}{500}$

   c $\dfrac{250}{1000}$

6 Multiply the following fractions

a $\dfrac{3}{6} \times \dfrac{18}{24}$

b $\dfrac{4}{12} \times \dfrac{16}{8}$

c $\dfrac{3}{9} \times \dfrac{24}{48}$

7 Divide the following fractions

a $\dfrac{10}{12} \div \dfrac{1}{4}$

b $\dfrac{1}{10} \div \dfrac{1}{50}$

c $\dfrac{1}{4} \div \dfrac{1}{100}$

8 Convert the following fractions to decimals

a $\dfrac{7}{10}$

b $\dfrac{5}{8}$

c $\dfrac{6}{40}$

9 Convert the following fractions to percentages

a $\dfrac{15}{20}$

b $\dfrac{7}{10}$

c $\dfrac{5}{8}$

10 Change the following decimals to fractions
   a 0.66
   b 0.1
   c 0.5

11 Change the following improper fractions to mixed fractions

   a $\dfrac{7}{4}$

   b $\dfrac{12}{5}$

   c $\dfrac{30}{7}$

12 Which of the following numbers will divide evenly into 75, 150, 300 respectively?
   a   (75)   2, 3, 5, 7, 15, 25
   b   (150)   4, 5, 6, 20, 30, 50
   c   (300)   2, 3, 5, 10, 25, 30, 50

13 Complete the following
   a   There are _____ mg in 6.5 g
   b   _____ mcg equals 1 g
   c   There are _____ cm in 1 m
   d   There are _____ m in 180 cm
   e   3.4 L equals _____ ml
   f   1 cc equals _____ ml

14 Convert the following
   a   1.25 mg to mcg
   b   2.5 L to ml
   c   0.65 g to mg
   d   1.6 m to cm
   e   375 ml to L
   f   75 cm to m

15 Express the following solute decimals as ratios _____ in _____
   a   0.75
   b   0.33
   c   0.4

16 Simplify the following ratios
   a   75 to 25
   b   50 in 150
   c   200 in 1000

17 Write as a percentage, the solutes for the given solvents
  a 80%
  b 35%
  c 95%

18 Change the following ratios ____ : ____ to ____ in ____
  a 2:3
  b 1:9
  c 4:6

ANSWERS

1 a 8499   **b** 3105   **c** 816.16   **d** 961.74

2 a 267   **b** 7096   **c** 676.6   **d** 582.2

3 a 133 776   **b** 14 322   **c** 64 280   **d** 46 900
   e 63 800   **f** 61.92   **g** 117.66

4 a 204   **b** 801   **c** 7.839   **d** 0.643
   e 46.8   **f** 60   **g** 650

5 a $\frac{2}{3}$ **b** $\frac{1}{5}$ **c** $\frac{1}{4}$

6 a $\frac{3}{8}$ **b** $\frac{2}{3}$ **c** $\frac{1}{6}$

7 a $3\frac{1}{3}$ **b** 5   **c** 25

8 a 0.7   **b** 0.625   **c** 0.15

9 a 75%   **b** 70%   **c** 62.5%

10 a $\frac{33}{50}$ **b** $\frac{1}{10}$ **c** $\frac{1}{2}$

11 a $1\frac{3}{4}$ **b** $2\frac{2}{5}$ **c** $4\frac{2}{7}$

12 a (75) 3, 5, 15, 25   **b** (150) 5, 6, 30, 50
   c (300) 2, 3, 5, 10, 25, 30, 50

13 a 6500   **b** 1 000 000   **c** 100   **d** 1.8
   e 3400   **f** 1

14	a	1250 mcg	b	2500 ml	c	650 mg	d	160 cm
	e	0.375 L	f	0.75 m				

15	a	3 in 4	b	1 in 3	c	2 in 5

16	a	3 to 1	b	1 in 3	c	1 in 5

17	a	20%	b	65%	c	5%

18	a	2 in 5	b	1 in 10	c	2 in 5

EXERCISE ONE

The first part of this book is a revision of the mathematics studied at school. You may need to revise some of these computations to enable you to move on and complete the following exercises.

ADDITION AND SUBTRACTION

When adding or subtracting numbers, it is important that the numbers are situated in such a way that the place value of each digit is adhered to.

 Example

28 + 317 + 26.4 + 18.2

Remember: 28 is actually 28.0

Decimal points need to be in line

```
   28.0
  317.0
   26.4
+  18.2
  389.6
```

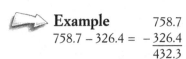 **Example**

$758.7 - 326.4 =$

```
  758.7
- 326.4
  432.3
```

Note: the decimal points are in line

Example

$$57.08 - 26 = \begin{array}{r} 57.08 \\ -\ 26.00 \\ \hline 31.08 \end{array}$$

 Activity

Add the following

1   **a** 20 + 46 + 83 + 174
     b 3 + 28 + 214 + 16
     c 1321 + 14 + 82 + 7
2   **a** 26.3 + 82.9 + 7.42
     b 85.23 + 12.1 + 6.86
     c 13.6 + 42.54 + 7.36
3   **a** 27 + 32.11 + 56.1
     b 38.2 + 14.9 + 28.34
     c 17.6 + 3.07 + 81

Subtract the following

4   **a** 7628 − 374
     b 2817 − 618
     c 784 − 632
5   **a** 965.02 − 36.1
     b 85.1 − 26.02
     c 369.74 − 82.07
6   **a** 264 − 82.06
     b 132.4 − 27.01
     c 485.37 − 28

MULTIPLICATION

 Example

2480 × 16 can be written as

$$\begin{array}{r} 2480 \\ \times\ 16 \\ \hline 14880 \\ 2480 \\ \hline 39680 \end{array}$$

Remember: keep the findings below the number that is multiplying. For example, you will note that $6 \times 0 = 0$, the zero is below the 6, as is the 0 from $1 \times 0 = 0$.

 Example

When multiplying any number by the power of 10, add one zero for each zero you are multiplying by.

600×10	becomes 6000 (one zero)
42×100	becomes 4200 (two zeros)
823×1000	becomes 823 000 (three zeros)

 Example

When a decimal point is involved during a multiplication by a power of 10, move the decimal point one place to the right for each zero involved.

5.82×10	becomes 58.2
0.46×100	becomes 46
1.62×1000	becomes 1620

 Example

When multiplying decimals, the number of digits after the decimal point in the answer must be equal to the total number of digits after the decimal points in the question.

2.4×0.73 is written as

$$
\begin{array}{r}
2.40 \\
\times\ 0.73 \\
\hline
720 \\
1680 \\
\hline
1.7520 \quad \text{or} \quad 1.752
\end{array}
$$

Note: the total of 4 digits after the decimal points, hence, there are 4 digits after the decimal point in the answer.

 Activity

Multiply the following

7   **a** 36×5
    b 147×22
    c 3608×123

8 a 7.4 × 8.6
   b 132.2 × 14.2
   c 872 × 17.14
9 a 8 × 18
   b 26 × 100
   c 132 × 1000
10 a 1.72 × 10
   b 23.1 × 100
   c 467.72 × 1000
11 a 49 × 7
   b 164 × 0.2
   c 0.25 × 6
12 a 0.001 × 1000
   b 0.68 × 100
   c 1.24 × 10
13 a 7.24 × 0.5
   b 328.01 × 10
   c 46.8 × 1000
14 a 0.75 × 0.5
   b 110 × 18.5
   c 0.75 × 60

DIVISION

Example
840 ÷ 4 can be written as

$$\begin{array}{r} 210 \\ 4\overline{)840} \end{array}$$

Note: 4 will divide into 8 twice (2 × 4 = 8), 4 will divide into 4 once, 4 will not divide into 0.

Example
50.65 ÷ 5 becomes

$$\begin{array}{r} 10.13 \\ 5\overline{)50.65} \end{array}$$

Note: 5 will divide into 5 once, 5 will not divide into 0, so write 0 and put the decimal point in place, 5 will divide into 6 once with 1 over making 5 into 15, 5 will divide into 15, 3 times.

Example

Division by the power of 10 requires the movement of the decimal
point one place to the left for each zero involved in the transaction.

84 ÷ 10	becomes	8.4
263 ÷ 100	becomes	2.63
1296 ÷ 1000	becomes	1.296
8.27 ÷ 10	becomes	0.827
16.4 ÷ 100	becomes	0.164
372.92 ÷ 1000	becomes	0.37292

 Activity

Divide the following

15 a 764 by 4
    b 1206 by 6
    c 936 by 3
    d 435 by 5
    e 729 by 9
    f 275 by 11
16 a 1008 by 10
    b 494 by 100
    c 792 by 1000
    d 678 by 100
    e 579 by 10
    f 864 by 1000

 Example

When the divisor (the number we are dividing by) is greater than 12,
it is easier to use the long division format to find the answer.
90 315 ÷ 15 can be written as

```
        06021
  15)90315
      90
      0031
        30
        15
        15
        00
```

Note: 15 into 9 will not divide, write zero. 15 into 90 will divide evenly 6 times. Bring down the 3 and place to the right of 00, 15 into 3 will not divide, write zero. Bring down the 1, making 31, 15 into 31 will divide twice with 1 over. Bring down the 5, making 15, 15 into 15 divides once, nothing remaining.

If the divisor contains a decimal point, the division cannot be completed until the decimal point has been moved. So, before beginning the division

- move the decimal point in the divisor to the right until it is no longer present
- remember, if the decimal point is moved one place to the right in the divisor, it must be moved one place to the right in the number being divided.

 ## Example

Mr Jones tells you that he weighs 9 stone 6 pounds and you are required to convert this weight to the metric format (in kilograms). You are aware that there are 14 pounds in each stone and that 2.2 pounds equals one kilogram. You convert his weight to pounds by multiplying 14 by 9 and adding the 6 pounds, making a total of 132 pounds. So, to find his weight in kg . . .

$$2.2\overline{)132}$$

Note: You need to move the decimal point in the divisor so that your calculation becomes 22 into 1320, 22 divides into 132, 6 times with nothing remaining. 22 will not divide into 0 so write 0.

$$\begin{array}{r} 60 \\ 22\overline{)1320} \\ \underline{132} \\ 00 \end{array}$$

His weight is 60 kg.

Activity

Divide the following

17 a 1008 by 14
    b 494 by 13
    c 792 by 22
    d 7.32 by 3
    e 48.04 by 4

18 a 1.2 by 10
    b 1.2 by 100
    c 1.2 by 1000
    d 845.7 by 100
    e 37.23 by 1000

19 a 396.12 by 3
    b 3315 by 195
    c 3245 by 25
    d 37.5 by 2.5
    e 145.2 by 2.2

20 a 14.6 by 10
    b 11.25 by 1000
    c 3245 by 100
    d 0.25 by 10
    e 1265 by 1000

EXERCISE TWO

FRACTIONS

A fraction is a numerical quantity that is not a whole number. It consists of a numerator (the top figure), a fraction bar (the divisor sign) and a denominator (the bottom figure). It should always be expressed in its lowest form.

Example

$\dfrac{6}{9} = \dfrac{2}{3}$ when cancelled down to its lowest form

This means that any number that will divide evenly into both the numerator and the denominator should be used to reduce the fraction to its lowest form. In this case, 3 went evenly into both 6 and 9.

An improper fraction is one where the numerator is greater than the denominator.

Example

$\dfrac{7}{4}$ can be converted to a mixed fraction by dividing the numerator (7) by the denominator (4).

$$4\overline{)7.0}^{\,1.75} \qquad \text{Note: } 1.75 = 1\dfrac{3}{4}$$

4 divides into 7 once with 3 left over. Thus, this mixed fraction is $1\dfrac{3}{4}$.

A mixed fraction can be converted to an improper fraction by multiplying the whole figure (1 in this case) by the denominator (4 in this case), then adding it to the numerator and dividing the total by the denominator.

 ## Example $\qquad\qquad 1 \times 4 + 3 \div 4 = \dfrac{7}{4}$

 ## Activity

Simplify the following fractions

1   a $\dfrac{64}{100}$

    b $\dfrac{10}{58}$

    c $\dfrac{7}{28}$

2   a $\dfrac{250}{1000}$

    b $\dfrac{1000}{4}$

    c $\dfrac{80}{100}$

3   a $\dfrac{1000}{8}$

   b $\dfrac{20}{60}$

   c $\dfrac{500}{4}$

4   a $\dfrac{250}{750}$

   b $\dfrac{125}{500}$

   c $\dfrac{125}{375}$

ADDITION AND SUBTRACTION OF FRACTIONS

To add or subtract fractions which have equal denominators, add or subtract the numerator.

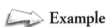 **Example** $\dfrac{3}{6} + \dfrac{2}{6}$ becomes $\dfrac{5}{6}$

                     $\dfrac{7}{8} - \dfrac{5}{8}$ becomes $\dfrac{2}{8}$ or $\dfrac{1}{4}$

If the denominators are not equal (suppose they are 3 and 7), before adding or subtracting the fraction, a denominator that is common to both figures (that is, both figures will divide evenly into this new figure) needs to be established. The fraction is then altered accordingly to maintain its quantity. 21 is the lowest common denominator (or the smallest number that they will both divide evenly into) for 3 and 7, hence it becomes the new denominator, but to keep the fraction constant, the numerator must be increased accordingly.

Example

$\dfrac{2}{3} - \dfrac{4}{7}$ becomes $\dfrac{2 \times 7}{3 \times 7} - \dfrac{4 \times 3}{7 \times 3}$ or $\dfrac{14}{21} - \dfrac{12}{21} = \dfrac{2}{21}$

With additions, the same principles apply.

Example

$$\frac{1}{2} + \frac{1}{3} \quad \text{becomes} \quad \frac{1 \times 3}{2 \times 3} + \frac{1 \times 2}{3 \times 2} \quad \text{or} \quad \frac{3}{6} + \frac{2}{6} = \frac{5}{6}$$

Activity

Subtract or add the following

5 **a** $\dfrac{2}{4} - \dfrac{1}{4}$

    b $\dfrac{1}{5} + \dfrac{7}{4}$

    c $\dfrac{11}{5} + \dfrac{2}{10}$

6 **a** $\dfrac{1}{2} + \dfrac{1}{4}$

    b $\dfrac{5}{8} - \dfrac{2}{4}$

    c $\dfrac{4}{9} - \dfrac{1}{3}$

7 Convert the following to improper fractions

    a $7\dfrac{2}{5}$

    b $3\dfrac{1}{4}$

    c $8\dfrac{1}{6}$

8 Convert the following to mixed fractions

    a $\dfrac{14}{3}$

    b $\dfrac{8}{5}$

    c $\dfrac{7}{2}$

MULTIPLICATION OF FRACTIONS

To multiply fractions, cancel any common factors which appear in the numerator and the denominator.

Multiply the numerators to obtain a numerator answer.
Multiply the denominators to obtain a denominator answer.
Check that the resulting fraction is expressed in its lowest form.

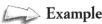 **Example**

$$\frac{2}{3} \times \frac{6}{8} \quad \text{becomes} \quad \frac{1}{1} \times \frac{2}{4} \quad \text{or} \quad \frac{1}{2}$$

2 divides into itself once and into 8 four times, 3 divides into itself once and into 6 twice

$$\frac{3}{7} \times \frac{4}{5} \quad \text{becomes} \quad \frac{3}{7} \times \frac{4}{5} \quad \text{or} \quad \frac{12}{35}$$

No digit will cancel down or divide evenly into any of the numbers, so multiply the top numbers and then the bottom ones

 Activity

Simplify or 'cancel down' the following fractions

9 a $\dfrac{3}{5} \times \dfrac{18}{24}$

b $\dfrac{3}{9} \times \dfrac{24}{48}$

c $\dfrac{4}{12} \times \dfrac{16}{8}$

10 a $\dfrac{1000}{5} \times \dfrac{15}{60}$

b $\dfrac{500}{5} \times \dfrac{12}{60}$

c $\dfrac{100}{2} \times \dfrac{14}{60}$

11 a $\dfrac{6}{10} \times \dfrac{1000}{4} \times \dfrac{25}{60}$

b $\dfrac{75}{100} \times \dfrac{500}{4} \times \dfrac{20}{60}$

c $\dfrac{20}{100} \times \dfrac{600}{3} \times \dfrac{15}{60}$

12 a $\dfrac{96}{48} \times \dfrac{200}{6} \times \dfrac{3}{9}$

b $\dfrac{18}{3} \times \dfrac{60}{4} \times \dfrac{7}{21}$

c $\dfrac{15}{60} \times \dfrac{500}{4} \times \dfrac{72}{100}$

DIVISION OF FRACTIONS

Where the division of a fraction is required, the divisor of the fraction is inverted and the computation is the same format as a multiplication.

 Example

$\dfrac{3}{4} \div \dfrac{1}{8}$ becomes $\dfrac{3}{4} \times \dfrac{8}{1}$ becomes $\dfrac{24}{4} = 6$

This computation could be used when preparing a weaker solution from a more concentrated solution. Suppose you needed to make up a 100 ml solution at 25% from a stock solution of 50%. Your first step would be to convert the percentages to fractions:

25% is $\dfrac{25}{100}$ and 50% is $\dfrac{50}{100}$

So, what you want is $\dfrac{25}{100} \div \dfrac{50}{100}$

This becomes $\dfrac{25}{100} \times \dfrac{100}{50}$ or $\dfrac{1}{2}$

In this case, half of the 100 ml solution or the solute will be the 50% solution and the other half will be the solvent, probably water.

Activity

Divide the following fraction and reduce your answer to the lowest common denominators

13 a $\dfrac{16}{20} \div \dfrac{1}{10}$

b $\dfrac{75}{50} \div \dfrac{1}{4}$

c $\dfrac{30}{60} \div \dfrac{3}{20}$

14 a $\dfrac{1}{4} \div \dfrac{1}{8}$

b $\dfrac{2}{3} \div \dfrac{1}{6}$

c $\dfrac{10}{12} \div \dfrac{1}{4}$

CONVERTING FRACTIONS TO DECIMALS

If you wish to convert a fraction to a decimal, you need to divide the denominator (the bottom number) into the numerator (the top number).

Example   Convert the fraction $\dfrac{2}{5}$ into a decimal

5 does not divide into 2 so write 0, add the decimal point and convert the 2 into 20, 5 divides into 20 four times.

Thus, $\dfrac{2}{5}$ becomes the decimal 0.4

Activity

Convert the following fractions into decimals. You may wish to simplify these fractions before you begin this task.

15 a $\dfrac{7}{10}$

b $\dfrac{1}{6}$

c $\dfrac{5}{12}$

d $\dfrac{3}{4}$

e $\dfrac{1}{2}$

f $\dfrac{1}{4}$

g $\dfrac{3}{5}$

h $\dfrac{1}{3}$

i $\dfrac{6}{10}$

CONVERTING FRACTIONS TO PERCENTAGES

A percentage is defined as the number of parts per hundred.

 Example   Convert $\dfrac{2}{5}$ to a percentage

It becomes $\dfrac{2}{5} \times \dfrac{100}{1} = 2 \times 20$ or 40%

 Activity

Convert the following fractions into percentages

16 a $\dfrac{13}{26}$

b $\dfrac{50}{100}$

c $\dfrac{2}{3}$

d $\dfrac{4}{10}$

e $\dfrac{1}{8}$

f $\dfrac{3}{9}$

g $\dfrac{75}{100}$

h $\dfrac{1}{2}$

17 Which of the following numbers will divide evenly into 150, 100, 75 respectively?
a (150)   2, 3, 5, 7, 10, 20, 25, 50
b (100)   2, 4, 5, 8, 10, 20, 25, 30
c (75)   2, 3, 5, 7, 9, 15, 20

Complete the following

18 a Remembering that each inch is equal to 2.54 cm, how many inches are there in 180 cm?
    b Each kilogram is equal to 2.2 pounds. How many pounds would a person weigh if his weight in kg was 60?
    c Convert to pounds, the weight of a child weighing 22 kilograms.

19 a Sally, who has just had her tonsils removed, is to have her orange juice diluted. She is to have 100 ml in total, and if 75% is fruit juice, how many ml of ice water will need to be added?
    b Tom is permitted 1500 ml of fluid per day. He is to have one third of this fluid before lunch. How many ml of fluid has he left for the remainder of the day?
    c Peter is to have a quarter of a tablet for an earache. If the whole tablet contains 500 mg, how many mg will he be given?

20 a You are to make up 200 ml of a medicated solution to clean a wound. If 5% of this solution is pure medication, how much sterile water will be required to complete the task?
    b Polly weighs 75 kilograms. She would like to lose a fifth of her body weight. How many kilograms will she need to lose?

c Polly is to have 1500 calories per day, two-thirds of which is to be complex carbohydrates. How many calories will be allocated to protein and fat?

EXERCISE THREE

Activity

Since you have become a university student who is studying for a degree in nursing, you have moved into a house which you share with two other girls. You are now considering the cost of this move.

1 Several expensive books are required to be purchased for this course. For example, you need a basic science book which is $42.60, an anatomy and physiology book which is $89.35, a nursing text for $78.90, law for nurses for $36.25, a bioethics text for $45.20 and a drug calculation workbook for $39.50. How much will it cost you to purchase these books?

2 Your parents gave you $350 for your books. Is there any change, and if so, how much?

3 You are fortunate to have a small casual job which begins in week one of the semester. In the first week you work 6.3 hours, in week three, you work 12.2 hours, week four, 4.5 hours and in week six, 7 hours. How many hours have you worked so far?

4 If your wage is $9.95 per hour, how much have you earned to date?

5 What is your average weekly wage for this six-week period?

6 Each week you must contribute $50 for the rent, $32.45 for food, $0.90 for electricity, $2.50 for the telephone, and $0.75 for the gas bill. Your parents have given you an allowance of $135 per week, so how much have you left after these bills have been paid?

7 If your average salary from the previous six weeks work continues, how much pocket money, in total, will you have for travelling and incidentals?

8 You purchase your lunch at the cafeteria each day and you usually buy a salad and ham roll for $3.50, a small chocolate bar for $1.25 and a 300 ml carton of flavoured milk for $1.60. However, you soon decide that university cafeteria meals are too expensive and plan to bring your own lunch.

   a You estimate that four slices of wholemeal bread will cost 40 cents, two slices of ham or other protein will cost 90 cents, a tomato will cost 60 cents and 500 ml of skim milk can be purchased for 65 cents. How much will your homemade lunch cost you?

   b If you attend university four days per week, what deductions will you need to make from your weekly pocket money to pay for your lunches?

   c Considering what you were paying for your lunch when you purchased it from the cafeteria, what savings are you making each week?

9 Train fares are $1.90 per day. How much would you expect to pay for your fares each week?

10 What will your fares cost for the thirteen-week semester?

11 How much rent will you pay each year?

12 If the telephone rental is $38 per quarter (= 13 weeks) and you are required to pay your share (one third), how much credit do you have for local calls each quarter?

13 If each local call costs 22 cents, how many local calls are you entitled to each quarter?

You are having great difficulties finding time to do all the things that you would like to do each week. Assignments are overdue and readings are behind schedule. You decide to work out a time management plan to help you to reach your goals.

14 Calculate the number of hours required each week for your university commitment if class attendance is 19 hours, lunch is 4 hours and travelling is 8 hours.

15 Taking into account the average number of hours that you work each week, what is your total commitment to work and study?

16 If, over the week, you plan to have 8 hours sleep each night, watch television for 8 hours and spend 5 hours on a recreational activity each week, how much time do you actually have left after work and university commitments are considered?

17 From the above figure you will need to take into account a further 36 hours for meals, housework and hygiene. So how much time is left to plan your studies?

18 As you attend university only four days per week, you decide that you will spend 10 hours of day five in preparation and for writing up assignments. How much time is left now?

19 If Sunday afternoon (from 13.00 to 18.00) is spent reading, in preparation for the following week, what remaining time could be allocated to revision on the four days you attend university?

20 Taking into account the time that you are spending on train journeys, are there any activities that could be carried out during this time, and if so, what and how much time could be saved for other activities?

EXERCISE FOUR

Activity

Mrs Smith, your neighbour, invites you to her place for afternoon tea and a chat. Because you are a nurse (albeit a very new one), she thinks that you will be able to answer all her questions!

1 She tells you that she has decided to lose weight and is very pleased with her progress. Before baby Peter was born she was 85.4 kg and now she is 71.7 kg. How much weight has she lost?

2 If the birth of baby Peter contributed to a loss of 12.5 kg, what is her actual weight loss?

3 She confides in you that she does not understand the metric system and asks you to convert her total loss to the 'old system' (the imperial system). You are aware that there are 2.2 pounds per kg, so what is her actual weight loss in pounds?

4 Mrs Smith tells you that she is having 7000 kilojoules each day, She asks you to convert this to calories because she is much more comfortable with that term. If each calorie is approximately 4 kilojoules (kj), what is her daily caloric intake?

5 10% of her diet is to be allocated to fat. How many calories can she set aside for fat?

6 If each gram of fat contains 9 calories, how many grams of fat can she have each day?

7 **a** The ideal body weight for her height is 60 kg. If she is permitted 0.75 grams of protein per kg of ideal body weight per day, how many grams can she have?
   b Because she is breast feeding, her protein intake can be increased to 1 gram/kilogram of ideal body weight. What % increase would this be?

8 If each gram of protein contains 4 calories, how many calories should be allocated to protein each day?

9 How many calories are left for her carbohydrate intake?

10 Of the remaining calories, two-thirds should be used for complex carbohydrates such as bread, cereal and rice. How many calories remain for simple carbohydrates, for example, sweets?

11 Mrs Smith says that the 'Baby Clinic' has told her to drink eight glasses, or 2 L of water each day to ensure a good supply of milk for Peter. She shows you her glass and you note that it holds 180 ml. Is she in fact having 2 L of water each day if she has eight drinks from this glass?

12 Mrs Smith tells you that she visited the baby clinic today to have a test weigh for Peter to see if he is receiving enough milk per feed. She says that Peter was 6.18 kg before his feed and he weighed 6.36 kg after the feed. What is his weight gain for this test feed?

13 If one gram of weight is equal to one ml of milk, how much milk did Peter have during that feed?

14 Mrs Smith says that Peter usually feeds every three hours but settles after his 9 pm feed and does not wake until 6 am. If his intake is constant, approximately how much milk does he receive each day?

15 Peter was 6.6 pounds when he was born and now he weighs 5.7 kg without his clothes. Taking into account that there are 2.2 pounds in every kilogram, how much weight has he gained?

16 Mrs Smith expresses her concerns about Robert, her five-year-old. She tells you that he will not eat properly and always has coughs and colds. He is 110 cm tall and weighs 18.5 kg. She asks you to convert his measurements to the imperial system.
   a Remembering that there are 2.54 cm to one inch, what is Robert's height in inches?
   b If there are 12 inches in each foot, what is his height in feet and inches?

17 **a** Taking into account that there are 2.2 pounds in each kilogram, what is his weight in pounds?
   b If there are 14 pounds in one stone, what is his weight in stones and pounds?

Mrs Smith brings you Robert's chest infection medications for inspection. She tells you that he is taking two tablets, three times each day. You are told that 36 tablets remain in the bottle and Robert needs to continue with this regime for another week. She asks you if she will need to get another prescription.

18 What advice should you give her?

19 If each tablet in the bottle contains 125 mg of medication, how many mg of this drug is Robert receiving each day?

20 She shows you a 100 ml bottle of medicine and says that Robert is to have 5 ml, three times each day. When she asks you how long she can expect the bottle to last, what should you tell her?

EXERCISE FIVE

Activity

As the first half of your semester finishes, you realise just how stressed you are. It is suggested that over the intra-semester break, you commence an exercise program to help you relax, keep fit and also to tone up your muscles. Investigation into what sorts of exercise programs are available in your community soon convinces you that devising your own program is not only the easiest but also the cheapest!

1 As part of your 'keep fit' plan, you decide to run seven laps around the oval three times per week. If each lap measures 560 metres (m), what distance will you run (in metres) each time?

2 If 1000 m equals one kilometre (km), what is the distance in km?

3 How many km will you run each week?

4 If you run at the rate of 10 km per hour, how long will each run last?

5 Running at the above speed utilises (approximately) 2400 kilojoules (kj) per hour. How many kj will you use up during this exercise program each week?

6 If 4 kilojoules equals approximately one calorie, what is the above measurement in calories?

7 If you are required to burn up 7000 calories to lose one kilogram of body fat, how long (in time) would you need to exercise at your present rate to lose 3 kg?

You soon decide that running alone is boring so you and your housemates visit the 'pound' and purchase a dog—which will also be useful in guarding your property! Being relatively poor, you decide to purchase the dog food in bulk.

8 The total cost of the dog food is $106.35. You have estimated an output of $5.75 per week and hope that the food will last sixteen weeks—will it?

9 The dog is more than happy to run with you three times each week, and your two housemates each offer to run two days per

week with the dog. If Jane does three laps around the oval, how far is that?

10 Sandy offers four laps per session. What is the total distance she will cover each week?

11 How many km will the dog run each week?

During the inter-semester break you are able to increase your casual work. In week one, you work 18.6 hours, week two, 23.4 hours, week three, 16.8 hours and in week four, 26 hours.

12 What is the total number of hours that you worked during these four weeks?

13 What is the average time that you spent working over these four weeks?

14 In relation to the previous average time spent working (5 hours/ week), what is the percentage increase in your work now?

15 If you were able to save one half of the money that you have just earned ($9.95 per hour) towards your uniforms, how much could you put aside for this purpose?

16 A visit to the uniform factory informs you that a shirt/top will cost you $29.50, slacks are $43.20 per pair, a jacket costs $59.95. How much will these articles cost in total?

17 You also need shoes which are $60.60, socks or stockings are $3.95 per pair, and a sleeveless vest for cooler days, which sells for $25.30. What will be the total cost for these items?

18 Having spoken to some second-year students you decide to purchase two tops, two pairs of slacks, two pairs of socks, a pair of shoes and a sleeveless vest. How much will this cost you?

19 Taking into account what you have saved towards your uniforms, will you need to ask your parents for extra money for these purchases, and if so, how much?

20 If you do not need assistance from your parents, how much money do you have in hand?

EXERCISE SIX

Activity

You have been allocated to your first clinical placement and it is situated 27 km from your residence. Your mother has very kindly offered to let you borrow her car should you wish to do so.

1 Your first placement is five days in a nursing home. How many km will you travel, in total, to meet this first commitment?

2 You have estimated that car costs will be 9.6 cents per kilometre for this placement. What is the cost per day?

3 What will be the total cost of petrol/car expenses for this placement?

4 It is soon apparent that, if you 'car pool', expenditure for travel will be reduced. You decide to share with three other students going to the same clinical venue. What will be the cost of travel for each student per day now?

5 What will be the cost of your travel for this placement if you 'car pool' for the last three days?

6 You purchase your lunch at a small café close to the nursing home. A sandwich with salad and ham costs $3.20, a small bottle of orange juice costs $1.20 and fruit is 50 cents. What will your five meals cost you for the week?

7 What will this placement cost you in relation to food and travel?

The next phase of your clinical placement is in a big city hospital just 5 km from your residence. For this two-week placement you are unable to 'car pool'. Should you make the decision to drive to this placement, you will need to spend $1.50 per hour for parking, and you will be expected to remain at the placement for eight hours each day.

8 Taking into account the cost of the petrol and the fees for parking, what will this placement cost you if you chose to drive?

9 The train fare is $1.90 each way or $9.50 per week if you purchase a weekly ticket. What would be the most economical means of travel for you over the two-week placement?

You decide to purchase a weekly train ticket, and in view of the fact that you need to leave home reasonably early to arrive at your destination by 07.00 sharp, you decide to continue to buy your lunch, this time at the hospital kiosk each day.

10 A small plate of salad costs 90 cents, cheese and crackers are $1.20, a piece of fruit costs 30 cents and a small carton of flavoured milk is $1.30. What will it cost you for lunches during this placement?

11 Including travel costs and meals, how much will this placement cost you?

Clinical experience for students is a valuable but a costly exercise. It costs the university $26.11 per hour for student supervision of approximately eight students in the first year.

12 How much per hour is this for each student?

13 What is the cost to the university for the three-week placement for you if you have eight-hour shifts each day?

14 What is the total cost for the eight students for the three weeks?

15 If the university sends out 384 students for a three-week placement in the first year, what is the expected cost if the ratio is one teacher to eight students?

If students miss practical experience due to illness, or for any other reason during their clinical placement, they may be required to 'make up' the missed time during the Christmas break. The clinical teacher, who supervises you while you are on placement, will be paid at the same rate whether she has six or eight students, so any time missed means that money paid to her loses its maximum potential.

16 Taking into account the hourly rate of pay for sessional teachers, what will it cost the taxpayer if you are required to make up 21 missed hours?

17 What would it cost the university if half of the first-year students had to make up two days each?

Following your successful clinical placement, you are offered a small part-time job in the nursing home where you did your first placement. You have been asked to work from 07.00 to 13.30 on Saturday mornings and from 13.00 to 19.30 on Sundays. Even though you only have a 30-minute break on each shift, and the work is quite tiring, you decide to accept the offer because you believe it will help you to develop your interpersonal and time management skills

18 Your salary for this experience will be $13.50 per hour. How much will you receive each week?

19 You have six weeks before semester ends and you expect to work December, January and February (13 weeks). How much could you expect to earn in this period?

20 Tax for this work will be $180. If you are able to save half of what you have earned to put towards your clinical placement in year two, how much will you have to spend over Christmas?

Having completed the exercises on basic mathematics, go to Practical Nursing Calculations website (see p. x) and complete Module One, Assessments One and Two. It is expected that your answers should be 100% correct to ensure your safety with the nursing calculations in the future.

If you are ready to move on, it is now time to commence the exercises related to the metric system in this workbook.

EXERCISE SEVEN

THE METRIC SYSTEM

The metric system is a system of measurement based on a decimal system that can be divided or multiplied by 10, 100, 1000 or 1 000 000. Prefixes are used in this system and are joined to the name of the primary or basic unit. They are the same throughout for weight, volume and length.

The basic units are metre, litre and gram. Prefixes in common use include

Micro	0.000001	or	one-millionth
Milli	0.001	or	one-thousandth
Centi	0.01	or	one-hundredth
Deci	0.1	or	one-tenth

Deka	10 ×	or	ten times as much
Hecto	100 ×	or	one hundred times as much
Kilo	1000 ×	or	one thousand times as much

When prefixes or units are written in full (for example, kilogram), they are usually written in lower case.

Symbols are used to represent prefixes and units. These symbols are internationally recognised representations and are *not* abbreviations of the unit names, thus they are *not* followed by full stops and they do not take a plural form.

 Example   kilogram is kg whether for one or three kilograms
Only one unit is used at a time.

 Example   3.6 kilometres is 3.6 km, *not* 3 km 600 m

Common terms in use

kilo	k
hecto	h
deka	da
deci	d
centi	c
micro	µ
metre	m
gram	g
milligram	mg
microgram	µg or mcg
litre	L (upper case to avoid confusion)
millilitre	ml or mL

Remember

1000 grams	= 1 kilogram
1000 milligrams	= 1 gram
1000 micrograms	= 1 milligram
1 000 000 micrograms	= 1 gram
100 centimetres	= 1 metre
10 millimetres	= 1 centimetre
1000 millilitres	= 1 litre
1 cc	= 1 ml = 1 g

Activity

Convert the following metric values

1 a 1 L to ml
   b 1 kg to g
   c 1 g to mg
   d 1 cm to mm

   e 1 g to mcg
   f 1 km to m
   g 1 m to cm
   h 1 mg to mcg

METRIC CONVERSION

This is the process by which the same quantity of a substance is described in a different term or unit. These equivalents are computed by:
- dividing, or moving the decimal point to the left, and
- multiplying, or moving the decimal point to the right.

Example

To change milligrams (a smaller unit) to grams (a larger unit), the milligrams are divided by 1000 (the number of milligrams in a gram). Therefore to express 50 mg in g, one needs to divide 50 by 1000, which becomes 0.05 g.

To change a larger unit (grams) to a smaller unit (milligrams), one needs to multiply. For example, to express 0.75g in mg, one needs to multiply 0.75 by 1000, which becomes 750 mg.

Activity

1 Change to litres
   a 750 ml
   b 15 ml
   c 3 ml

2 Change to millilitres
   a 0.72 L
   b 1.06 L
   c 0.004 L

3 Change to metres
   a 67 cm
   b 184 cm
   c 30 cm

4 Change to centimetres
  a 0.8 m
  b 2.45 m
  c 0.01 m

5 Change to millilitres
  a 1.6 L
  b 0.4 L
  c 10 L

6 Change to grams
  a 1.24 kg
  b 0.91 kg
  c 0.06 kg

7 Change to milligrams
  a 2.5 g
  b 0.6 g
  c 0.002 g

8 Change to grams
  a 600 mg
  b 64 mg
  c 5 mg

9 Change to micrograms
  a 1.5 mg
  b 0.65 mg
  c 0.1 mg

Convert the following
10 **a** 0.4 L to ml
    b 750 mg to g
    c 1 500 000 mcg to g

11 **a** 0.25 mg to mcg
    b 1.25 g to mcg
    c 150 cm to m

12 **a** 1 g to mg
    b 1 mg to g
    c 1 mg to mcg

13 **a** 10 cm to m

    b 1.5 m to cm

    c 15 mm to cm

14 **a** 15 ml to L

    b 4.5 L to ml

    c 750 ml to L

15 **a** 0.4 mg to mcg

    b 600 mcg to mg

    c 75 mg to g

16 **a** 650 mcg to mg

    b 0.5 g to mg

    c 6 ml to L

17 **a** You are caring for a frail, elderly man whose wife tells you that he is 7 stone 6 pounds. Remembering that there are 14 pounds in one stone and 2.2 pounds to a kg, covert his weight to kg.

    b She says that he is 5 feet 10 inches tall. Remembering that there are 12 inches to a foot, and that 2.54 cm make one inch, convert his height to cm.

    c Convert his height to metres.

18 **a** This frail, elderly man is having 2 g of drug A each day, in four equally divided doses. How many mg will he have with each dose?

    b He also has 125 mg of drug B every 4 hours. Write his daily dose in grams.

    c Drug C is available in 0.5 g tablets and he is to have 250 mg per dose. How many tablets should he be given?

19 **a** This gentleman has a chest infection and you are to encourage him to drink a lot of fluid. He is to have a minimum of 1.5 L each day. How many ml would this be?

    b You have been asked to give him small drinks frequently. If you gave him a drink every hour, on the hour, from 09.00 to 18.00 inclusive, how many drinks will he have?

    c To reach the minimum target of 1.5 L, how much fluid should you offer him per drink?

EXERCISE EIGHT

Activity

You are caring for Peter Jones, a young man with a chest infection. He has been ordered 3 mg of drug A per kilogram of body weight per day. He weighs 70 kg.

1   **a** How many mg of drug A will he have each day?
    b If this medication is to be given in three equally divided doses, how many mg should he receive per dose?
    c Write a single dose in grams.

2   Drug B is to be given every 4 hours. He is to have 150 mg per dose. How many mg will he have in a 24-hour period?

Drug C is ordered for his cough. This cough mixture has a concentration of 50 mg per ml of fluid. Peter is to have 2.5 grams of this medicated solution each day, in five equally divided doses.

3   **a** How many mg per dose should he have?
    b What volume of medicine is needed for a single dose?

4   **a** The medication for his cough (drug C) is available in a 0.5 L bottle. How many ml would be in this bottle?
    b Taking into account the number of doses ordered each day and the volume of each dose, how long would you expect this bottle to last?

5   **a** Peter has an elevated temperature. Using the chart at the end of this exercise, identify the time and date of Peter's highest reading.
    b What is the temperature range for Peter during this period?

6   On the chart provided, demonstrate how you would chart Peter's 4-hourly pulse readings for the past four days. Day 1: 120, 124, 110, 122, 120, 118; Day 2: 116, 120, 110, 108, 120, 100; Day 3: 90, 96, 88, 74, 70, 68; Day 4: 62, 88, 90, 72, 70, 68.

7   Using the same chart, document his blood pressure for the past four days. Day 1: 140/90, 135/85; Day 2: 130/60, 135/65; Day 3: 125/60, 130/65; Day 4: 120/60, 125/75.

8   You are asked to encourage Peter to drink. If he drinks 0.2 L every hour for the next 10 hours, how much fluid (in total) will be charted on his fluid balance chart?

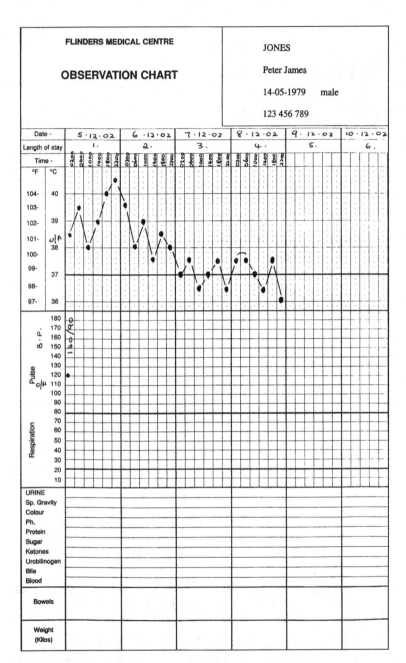

Figure 1.1

9 Tom Smith, in the bed next to Peter, has Diabetes and an infected leg ulcer. Twice each day, he has the equivalent of 0.5 g of drug A to help control his Diabetes. How many mg per dose is he receiving?

He also has an antibiotic injection to help to control the infection in his ulcer. The label on the bottle indicates that there are 250 mg of drug B in every ml of fluid.

10 **a** How many ml are there in the bottle if it contains 1 gram?
   b If Tom is to have 500 mg of this antibiotic every 4 hours, how many ml of fluid would each injection contain?
   c How many grams of this medication is Tom receiving each day?

Tom's leg ulcer is cleaned with a 10% solution of drug C. The total volume of this medicated solution is 20 ml.

11 **a** What volume of the 20 ml is actually drug C?
   b Drug C is the solute. Remembering that a solution is the solute + the solvent, what volume will be solvent?

12 **a** You are to make Tom a jug of diabetic cordial. He tells you to pour 150 ml of cordial into his 1 L jug. What volume of iced water is required to fill the 1 L jug?
   b Write the solute and solvent of this cordial-making exercise as a ratio, ___to___.
   c Convert the above ratio to a fraction and express it in its most simple form.

Tom is currently having all his fluid intake and output documented on a fluid balance chart. His daily intake for the day is: tea, 6 cups of 180 ml; soup, 200 ml; diabetic jelly, 0.15 L and diabetic cordial, 1.5 L. He has passed urine four times, 350 ml, 280 ml, 410 ml and 360 ml.

13 **a** What is his intake of fluid and his output for the day?
   b When you consider that his insensible loss (from breathing and perspiration) is approximately 600 ml, is his fluid balance negative (output more than intake) or positive (intake greater than output)?

Mr Bill Evans is also being nursed in the same bay. He was admitted because he had a heart condition that was unstable.

14 Mr Evans is to have 250 mcg of drug A to improve his heart contractions. The tablets in the ward are 0.25 mg. How many tablets should he be given?

15 Drug B is to help him rid his body of accumulating fluid. This medication is available as 40 mg tablets. If he is to have 80 mg, how many tablets should he be given?

16 Another tablet has been ordered to balance the salts in his body. He is to have 0.6 g of this medication. Stock available is 600 mg tablets. How many tablets should he be given?

17 His blood pressure has been higher than normal, so he has been ordered drug D to assist in lowering it. This tablet is available as a 30 mg tablet but he requires only 15 mg, so what should be given?

18 Another medication has been ordered to assist his circulation. He is to have 0.9 g per day in three equally divided doses. If the tablets available are 150 mg, how many should he be given for his 08.00 dose?

19 A fluid restriction is in place for this gentleman, permitting him 1.5 L per day. If his waking hours are from 07.00 to 22.00, how much fluid (on average) should he have per hour?

20 He asks for a sleeping tablet at night and is permitted 10 mg. If stock available is 5 mg tablets, how many should he be given?

EXERCISE NINE

Activity

Ms Jenny Lee has been admitted to hospital for investigation of abdominal pain. She weighs 75 kg.

1 Jenny is to have 3 mcg of drug A per kg of body weight per minute. How much of this medication will she receive every hour?

2 Write the above dose in milligrams.

3 What would be her daily dose of this medication in grams?

4   Drug B is to be given according to her body surface area (BSA). For each dose she is to have 2.5 mg per m^2 of body surface area. If her body surface area is 1.65 m^2, how much medication will be given per dose?

5   What is her daily requirement of drug B if she is to have this medication every four hours?

6   Jenny has a 500 ml bottle of mixture which contains 10 grams of drug C. How many mg of drug C is in one ml of this mixture?

7   Each dose of this mixture that Jenny receives is to contain 300 mg of drug C. How many ml would contain this dose?

8   If Jenny is to have this mixture three times each day, write her daily dose of this medication in grams.

Sometimes when people are admitted to hospital, it is necessary to measure the amount of fluid that they take into their bodies and the amount of fluid that leaves their bodies. There are several ways to record a person's intake and output and this will depend on the health agency that you are working for.

For this exercise, using the chart attached (see Fig. 1.2), all fluid that is offered is written in the 'oral' column and only what is actually consumed is written in the 'amount given' column. Using the following information, complete Jenny's fluid balance chart for day two.

• At midnight or 00.00 she had 360 ml of cordial in her water jug. She drank 100 ml at 06.00 with her medication. Her jug was removed and replaced with 1 L of fresh water at 07.00. She finished this jug at 14.00 and it was refilled with 1 L of fluid. At 24.00 220 ml remained in the jug.
• Throughout the day several cups of tea (150 ml) were offered. At 07.00, 10.00, 15.00, 20.00 she finished the tea but at 13.00 and 17.00, she drank only half of what was offered.
• She finished her 200 ml of soup at 12.00 and ate her jelly (150 ml) at 17.00.
• Unfortunately she vomited at 11.00 (300 ml) and again at 20.00 (250 ml).

		FLINDERS MEDICAL CENTRE	Ward	
		FLUID BALANCE CHART	Surname	LEE
			Other Names	Jenny Heather
			D.O.B./Sex	30-11-1980 female
Medical Officer:	Date:		Address	
			Medi. No.	987 654 321

	INTAKE				OUTPUT				
Time	By Mouth or Tube (Description)	ml	Intravenous	ml	Vomitus or Aspirate	ml	Faeces and Other Drainage (Description)	ml	Urine ml
0100									
0200									
0300									
0400									
0500									
0600									
0700									
0800									
0900									
1000									
1100									
1200									
1300									
1400									
1500									
1600									
1700									
1800									
1900									
2000									
2100									
2200									
2300									
2400									
Total..................									

Grand Total........   Grand Total........

(Not Including Insensible Loss)

Plus

Balance............................

Total Volume of
Blood Infused..   Minus

Figure 1.2

- Jenny voided 430 ml at 06.00, 300 ml at 09.00, 150 ml at 17.00 and 300 ml at 21.00.

9 a Total her intake and output on the chart provided.
   b Her insensible loss (via her breathing and perspiration) is considered to be 600 ml. When you take this into account, is her balance negative or positive?

10 Jenny is pregnant. If the birth of her baby is due 9 months and 7 days following the onset of her last menstrual period (2 March), when is her baby due?

11 Jenny is febrile (she has a temperature). On the chart provided (Fig. 1.3), record her temperature (every 4 hours) for the last 24 hours, beginning at 02.00: 39.0, 37.6, 38.2, 38.9, 37.8, 39.5.

12 Record her pulse (every 4 hours) for the same period, in the space provided: 110, 94, 98, 102, 96, 116.

Because Jenny continues to be nauseous (she feels sick), she is only to have clear fluids for the time being. She asks you to make her a jug of weak apple juice from the tin of pure juice that she has in her locker. She wants you to make up 0.5 L of drink, using the 300 ml tin.

13 Write the above dilution as a ratio _____ in _____. Simplify if necessary.

At 13.00, an intravenous infusion is commenced to ensure that Jenny is receiving enough fluid. She has a 1 L bag of 0.9% sodium chloride.

14 a How many ml of fluid is in 1 L?
   b If this 1 L bag is to last for 10 hours, how much fluid should Jenny receive from her intravenous every hour?

At 16.00, Jenny's condition has not improved, she is still quite nauseated and has vomited 200 ml of the diluted apple juice. A decision is made to increase her intravenous fluid intake.

15 How much fluid has Jenny received from her intravenous infusion so far?

16 Approximately 690 ml remain in the bag. Has this been dripping to schedule?

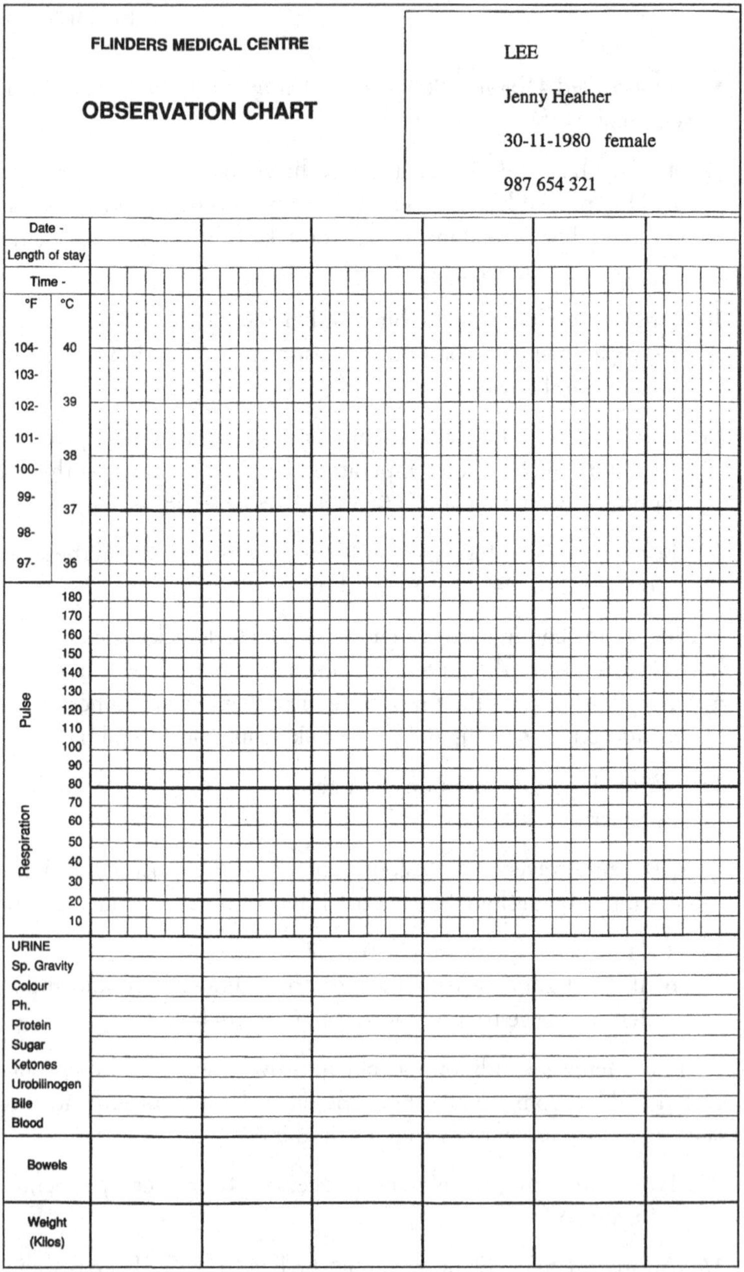

FLINDERS MEDICAL CENTRE	LEE
OBSERVATION CHART	Jenny Heather
	30-11-1980 female
	987 654 321

Date -	
Length of stay	
Time -	

°F	°C
104-	40
103-	
102-	39
101-	
100-	38
99-	
98-	37
97-	36

Pulse

180
170
160
150
140
130
120
110
100
90
80
70
60
50
40
30
20
10

Respiration

URINE
Sp. Gravity
Colour
Ph.
Protein
Sugar
Ketones
Urobilinogen
Bile
Blood
Bowels
Weight (Kilos)

Figure 1.3

17 If the remaining 690 ml in to infuse in 4 hours, how many ml per hour should Jenny now receive?

18 How many ml per minute should she receive?

19 Every ml of intravenous fluid that Jenny receives is made up of 20 drops that pass through the transparent chamber on the intravenous set, so how many drops per minute should she receive?

20 Construct a formula to determine the number of drops of intravenous fluid/minute for a person receiving 200 ml over 2 hours if the drop factor for the giving set is 20 drops/ml.

EXERCISE TEN

SOLUTIONS

A solution is a mixture that contains one or more substances dissolved in it.

$$\text{solution} = \text{solute} + \text{solvent}$$

The solute is the substance that is dissolved in the fluid and the solvent is the fluid in which the solute is dissolved. The substances (solutes) may be dry as sugar in a cup of coffee or even the antibiotic powder that can be made up to form an injectable solution; or wet, as when making up a jug of cordial from a concentrated solution.

Dry substances are measured in weight and expressed as weight per volume (W/V) and fluid substances are measured in volume and expressed as volume per volume (V/V). It is important to remember that dry substances displace fluid when making up a solution.

RATIOS

A ratio is a comparison of two numbers, which can be written as a fraction, a decimal, a percentage, or by using a colon between two figures.

When a solution is described it has two or more parts; the solute is the proportion combined with the solvent to form the solution.

Example

You are to dilute (make up) some cordial for a child using a 25% solute. This could be expressed as 1 to 3 or 1 in 4 or 1:3.

1 part (solute) to 3 parts (solvent) = 4 parts (solution).

Make up 100 ml of cordial with a solute ratio of 1 to 3.
1 to 3 is also 1 in 4 which can be written as a fraction 1 ÷ 4.

 Formula

$$\frac{\text{Want}}{\text{Have}} \times \frac{\text{Amount required}}{1} \quad \text{or} \quad \times \frac{100}{1} = 25 \text{ ml solute, } 75 \text{ ml solvent}$$

Thus, you will combine 25 ml of cordial with 75 ml of water.

In most large city hospitals, solutions come to the wards already prepared at the required concentration, but in smaller country hospitals, where solutions can be quite concentrated and sometimes in their pure form, it could be your responsibility as the nurse, to further dilute the concentrate for use.

 Example

You are to make up 4 L of Sodium Hypochlorite (Milton's solution) to disinfect the baby's milk bottles. The strength required is 1 in 80.
Make up 4000 ml of a 1 in 80 concentration (solution).

$$\frac{1}{80} \times \frac{4000}{1} = \frac{400}{8} \text{ or } 50 \text{ ml solute}$$

Thus, you will combine 50 ml of Sodium Hypochlorite with 3950 ml of tap water to form the required concentration.

At times, the stock available is not in its pure format. For example, it may have a concentration of 20% and you are required to make up a solution of 10%.

Example

You need a 10% solution and the only available stock is 25%. In this case you will need to convert the percentages to fractions and divide what you want by what you have.

Make up 200 ml of 10% solution from a stock solution of 25%.

$$\frac{10}{100} \div \frac{25}{100} \times \frac{200}{1} \quad \text{becomes} \quad \frac{10}{100} \times \frac{100}{25} \times \frac{200}{1}$$

When the above equation is simplified you end up with the number 80. Thus, 80 ml of the 25% solute is combined with 120 ml of sterile water to achieve the desired concentration rate of 10%.

Should you be asked to make up 100 ml of solution with a 20% solute, the formula would be

$$\frac{20}{100} \; (20\% \text{ solute}) \times \frac{100}{1} \; (\text{volume in ml})$$

When cancelled down, 20 ml is solute and 80 ml is solvent; this simplified is 1 to 4. Remember, a 20% solution is 20 grams in 100 ml.

 Activity

1 Express the following solute ratios as fractions. Simplify where necessary
   a 1 in 2
   b 6 to 4
   c 3 to 7
   d 1 in 10

2 Express the following solute ratios as decimals
   a 4 in 10
   b 2 to 6
   c 2 in 5
   d 5 to 15

3 Express the following solute ratios as percentages
   a 100 in 1000
   b 30 to 70
   c 3 to 7
   d 15 in 100

4 Simplify the following ratios
   a 3 in 9
   b 8 to 12
   c 4 in 10
   d 2 in 10

5 Express the following solute percentages as ratios ___ to ___, simplify as required
   a 16%
   b 28%
   c 75%
   d 50%

6 Simplify the following ratios
   a 200 to 800
   b 15 to 85
   c 20 in 100
   d 40 in 60

7 Express the following solute decimals as ratios ___ in ___, simplify as required
   a 0.875
   b 0.66
   c 0.75
   d 0.5

8 Simplify the following ratios
   a 16 to 4
   b 18 in 72
   c 20 in 100
   d 10 to 90

9 Express the following solute fractions as ratios ___ to ___
   a 1/6
   b 3/8
   c 6/10
   d 2/6

10 Simplify the following ratios
   a 60 to 40
   b 12 in 36

   c 15 in 20

   d 12 to 24

11 A diluted substance has a strength (concentration) of 5 in 100. Express this as a ratio of concentrate to water.

12 A mixture contains 20 g of powder to 80 ml of water. Express this as a ratio of powder to water (W/V).

13 100 ml of solution contains 65 ml of solvent. What % of this solution is solute?

14 You are to make up 1 L of cordial with a 1 to 4 ratio of solute. How much water is required to complete this task?

15 A sick infant is to have diluted cows milk. Make up 200 ml of diluted milk with a 4 in 5 solute ratio indicating the amount of milk and water required for the task.

16 Pure apple juice is to be diluted with a ratio of 7 to 3. How much drink will the child have if the apple juice required is 70 ml?

17 You are to clean the dressing trolley with a 4% solution. Stock available is 6%. Make up 60 ml of 4% solution.

18 1 L of normal saline (0.9% sodium chloride) contains 0.9% solute. How many grams of salt (sodium chloride) would be in this solution?

19 How much dextrose would be in 1 L of a 5% solution?

20 The Arts Department has 35 male students and 155 female students. What is the ratio of female to male students?

Having completed all of the above exercises, go to the Practical Nursing Calculations website (see p. x) and complete Module One, Assessments Three and Four. Allow yourself 20 minutes for each assessment and, again, it is important that you get *all* computations correct.

When 100% pass has been achieved, move on to Module Two, which should coincide with the commencement of semester two, year one, of your undergraduate nursing degree.

ANSWERS

EXERCISE ONE

1	a	323	**b**	261	**c**	1424		
2	a	116.62	**b**	104.19	**c**	63.5		
3	a	115.21	**b**	81.44	**c**	101.67		
4	a	7254	**b**	2199	**c**	152		
5	a	928.92	**b**	59.08	**c**	287.67		
6	a	181.94	**b**	105.39	**c**	457.37		
7	a	180	**b**	3234	**c**	443 784		
8	a	63.64	**b**	1877.24	**c**	14 946.08		
9	a	144	**b**	2600	**c**	132 000		
10	a	17.2	**b**	2310	**c**	467 720		
11	a	343	**b**	32.8	**c**	1.5		
12	a	1	**b**	68	**c**	12.4		
13	a	3.62	**b**	3280.1	**c**	46 800		
14	a	0.375	**b**	2035	**c**	45		
15	a	191	**b**	201	**c**	312	**d**	87
	e	81	**f**	25				
16	a	100.8	**b**	4.94	**c**	0.792	**d**	6.78
	e	57.9	**f**	0.864				
17	a	72	**b**	38	**c**	36	**d**	2.44
	e	12.01						
18	a	0.12	**b**	0.012	**c**	0.0012	**d**	8.457
	e	0.03723						
19	a	132.04	**b**	17	**c**	129.8	**d**	15
	e	66						
20	a	1.46	**b**	0.01125	**c**	32.45	**d**	0.025
	e	1.265						

EXERCISE TWO

1 a $\dfrac{16}{25}$ b $\dfrac{5}{29}$ c $\dfrac{1}{4}$

2 a $\dfrac{1}{4}$ b 250   c $\dfrac{4}{5}$

3 a 125   b $\dfrac{1}{3}$ c 125

4 a $\dfrac{1}{3}$ b $\dfrac{1}{4}$ c $\dfrac{1}{3}$

5 a $\dfrac{1}{4}$ b $\dfrac{39}{20}$ c $\dfrac{12}{5}$

6 a $\dfrac{3}{4}$ b $\dfrac{1}{8}$ c $\dfrac{1}{9}$

7 a $\dfrac{37}{5}$ b $\dfrac{13}{4}$ c $\dfrac{49}{6}$

8 a $4\dfrac{2}{3}$ b $1\dfrac{3}{5}$ c $3\dfrac{1}{2}$

9 a $\dfrac{9}{20}$ b $\dfrac{1}{6}$ c $\dfrac{2}{3}$

10 a 50   b 20   c $11\dfrac{2}{3}$

11 a $62\dfrac{1}{2}$ b $31\dfrac{1}{4}$ c 10

12 a $22\dfrac{2}{9}$ b 30   c $22\dfrac{1}{2}$

13 a 8   b 6   c $3\dfrac{1}{3}$

14 a 2   b 4   c $3\dfrac{1}{3}$

15 a 0.7   b 0.166   c 0.416   d 0.75
    e 0.5   f 0.25   g 0.6   h 0.33
    i 0.6

16 a 50%   b 50%   c 66.66%   d 40%
    e 12.5%   f 33.33%   g 75%   h 50%

17 a 2, 3, 5, 10, 25, 50   b   2, 4, 5, 10, 20, 25   c   3, 5, 15

18 a 70.86 inches   b 132 lbs   c 48.4 pounds or 48 lb 6 oz

19 a 25 ml $\dfrac{75}{100} \times \dfrac{100}{1}$ = 75 ml orange juice + 25 ml of water

    b 1000 ml $\dfrac{1}{3} \times \dfrac{1500}{1}$ = 500 ml before lunch leaving 1000 ml for the rest of the day

    c 125 mg $\dfrac{1}{4} \times \dfrac{500}{1}$ = 125 mg

20 a 190 ml $\dfrac{5}{100} \times \dfrac{200}{1}$ = 10 ml of medicated solution + 190 ml of sterile water

    b 15 kg $\dfrac{1}{5} \times \dfrac{75}{1}$ = 15 kg to lose making her desired weight 60 kg

    c 500 $\dfrac{2}{3} \times \dfrac{1500}{1}$ = 1000 calories for carbohydrates and 500 for protein & fat

EXERCISE THREE

1 $331.80

2 Yes, $18.20

3 30 hours

4 $298.50

5 $49.75

6 $48.40

7 $98.15

8 a $2.55   b $10.20   c $15.20

9 $7.60

10 $98.80

11 $2600

12 $19.84

13 Approximately 90

14 31 hours

15 36 hours

16 63 hours

17 27 hours

18 17 hours

19 12 hours or 3 hours/day

20 8 hours travelling—use the time (approx 4–6 hours) for reading or revision

EXERCISE FOUR

1	13.7 kg	85.4 – 71.7
2	1.2 kg	13.7 – 12.5
3	2.64 pounds or 2 lb 10 oz	1.2 × 2.2
4	1750 calories	7000 ÷ 4
5	175	1750 ÷ 10
6	Approx 19–20	175 ÷ 9
7	**a** 45 g	60 kg × 0.75 g of protein
	b 25%	
8	240 calories	60 g of protein × 4 calories/gram
9	1335 calories	1750 – 175 – 240
10	Approx 445 calories	1/3 of 1335 = 444.9
11	No, she is only having 1.44 L	180 × 8
12	0.18 kg or 180 g	
13	180 ml	
14	1080 ml or 1.08 L	180 ml × 6 feeds
15	2.7 kg	6.6 ÷ 2.2 = 3; 5.7 – 3

16 a 43.3 inches   110 ÷ 2.54 cm/inch

    b 3 feet 6 inches (approx)   43.3 ÷ 12

17 a 40.7 pounds or 40 lb 11 oz   18.5 kg × 2.2 lb/kg

    b 2 stone 12 pounds 11 ounces   40.7 ÷ 14

18 Only enough for 6 days, will need another script

19 750 mg   125 mg × 6 doses

20 6 days and 2 doses   100 ÷ (3 × 5)

EXERCISE FIVE

1 3920 m   560 × 7

2 3.92 km

3 11.76 km   3.92 × 3

4 23.52 minutes   3.92 km × 6 minutes (1 km run/6 minutes)

5 2822 kj/week   2400 kj/hour = 40 kj/minute

                                     23.52 minutes × 3 times/wk = 70.56 mins

                                     70.56 minutes × 40 kj/minute = 2822

6 705 (approx)   2822 kj ÷ 4 kj/calorie = 705.5

7 35 hours   21 000 calories needed to lose 3 kg

                                     2400 kj/hour = 600 calories

                                     21 000 calories ÷ 600 calories = 35 hours

8 Yes $106.35 ÷ $5.75 = 18.49 weeks

9 1680 m   560 × 3

10 4480 m $\qquad$ 560 × (4 × 2)

11 19.6 km/week $\qquad$ 4.48 km + 3.36 km +
11.76 km

12 84.8 hours

13 21.2 hours/week $\qquad$ 84.8 ÷ 4

14 76.4% increase $\qquad$ 21.2 − 5 = 16.2

$$\frac{16.2}{21.1} \times \frac{100}{1} \text{ becomes } \frac{162}{212} \times \frac{100}{1}$$

15 $421.88 $\qquad$ 84.8 hours × $9.95 ÷ 2

16 $132.65

17 $89.85

18 $239.20

19 No, you should have enough money

20 $182.68

EXERCISE SIX

1 270 km

2 $5.18

3 $25.90

4 $1.30 (approx)

5 $14.26

6 $24.50

7 $38.76

8 $129.60 $\qquad$ 10 km at 9.6 cents/km ×
10 days = $9.60
$1.50 × 8 hrs × 10 days
= $120

9 By train $\qquad$ 2 × $9.50 tickets

10 $37

11 $56

12 $3.26/hour/student $26.11/hour ÷ 8 students

13 $391.20/student/placement $3.26/hr × 8 hours
                                                        = $26.08

                                                        $26.08/day × 15 days
                                                        = $391.20

14 $3129.60 $391.20 × 8 students

15 $150 220.80   384 ÷ 8 = 48 weeks ×
                                                        $3129.60

16 $68.46 $3.26 × 21 hours

17 $10 014.72   1/2 = 192 students; 192 ×
                                                        $26.08 × 2 days

18 $162   Sat + Sun = 12 hours at
                                                        $13.50

19 $3078 $162/week × 19 weeks

20 $1449 $3078 – $180 = $2898 ÷ 2

EXERCISE SEVEN

1	**a** 1000	**b** 1000	**c** 1000	**d** 10			
	e 1 000 000	**f** 1000	**g** 100	**h** 1000			

2 a 0.75   b 0.015   c 0.003

3 a 720   b 1060   c 4

4 a 0.67   b 1.84   c 0.3

5 a 80   b 245   c 1

6 a 1600   b 400   c 10 000

7 a 1240   b 910   c 60

8 a 2500   b 600   c 2

9 a 0.6   b 0.064   c 0.005

10 a 1500   b 650   c 100

11   **a** 400   **b** 0.75   **c** 1.5

12   **a** 250   **b** 1 250 000   **c** 1.5

13   **a** 1000   **b** 0.001   **c** 1000

14   **a** 0.1   **b** 150   **c** 1.5

15   **a** 0.015   **b** 4500   **c** 0.75

16   **a** 400   **b** 0.6   **c** 0.075

17   **a** 0.65   **b** 500   **c** 0.006

18   **a** 47.27 kg $14 \times 7 + 6 = 104 \div 2.2$
     b 177.8 cm $5 \times 12 + 10 = 70 \times 2.54$
     c 1.78 m (approx)

19   **a** 500 mg/dose $2 \text{ g} = 2000 \text{ mg} \div 4 \text{ doses}$
     b 0.75 grams $125 \text{ mg} \times 6 \text{ doses} \div 1000$
     c 1/2 tablet $250 \div 500 = 0.5$

20   **a** 1500 ml
     b 10 drinks
     c 150 ml/drink $1500 \text{ ml} \div 10 \text{ drinks}$

EXERCISE EIGHT

1   **a** 210 mg/day $3 \text{ mg} \times 70 \text{ kg}$
     b 70 mg/dose $210 \text{ mg} \div 3 \text{ doses}$
     c 0.07 grams

2   900 mg $150 \text{ mg/dose} \times 6 \text{ doses}$

3   **a** 500 mg $2500 \text{ mg} \div 5 \text{ doses}$
     b 10 ml/dose $500 \text{ mg} \div 50 \text{ mg/ml}$

4   **a** 500 ml
     b 10 days   5 doses of 10 ml/dose =
                                 50 ml/day
                                 $500 \text{ ml} \div 50 \text{ ml/day} = 10$

5   **a** 22.00, 5.12.02
     b 36°C to 40.5°C

6   See Figure 1.4

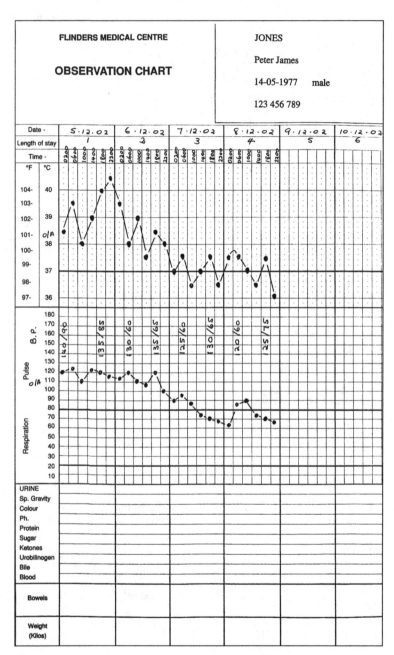

Figure 1.4

7 See Figure 1.4

8 2 litres

9 500 mg/dose

10 a 4 ml   1000 mg ÷ 250 mg/ml
   b 2 ml   1 ml = 250 mg, so 500 mg
                                     = 2 ml

   c 3 grams   500 mg/dose × 6 doses

11 a 2 ml $\dfrac{10}{100} \times \dfrac{20}{1} = 2$

   b 18 ml   20 ml of solution – 2 ml of
                                     solute

12 a 850 ml   1000 ml – 150 ml cordial (solute)
   b 150 to 850

   c $\dfrac{3}{17}$ Cancel down the 150 & 850

13 a 2930 ml, 1400 ml
   b 930 ml, positive   2930 ml in & 2000 ml out
                                     = +930 ml

14 1 tablet   0.25 mg = 250 mcg

15 2 tablets

16 1 tablet   0.6 g = 600 mg

17 1/2 tablet

18 2 tablets   0.9 g = 900 mg ÷ 3 doses of
                                   300 mg; each tablet is 150 mg
                                   so 2 tabs needed

19 100 ml/hour   1500 ml ÷ 15 hours

20 2 tablets   each tablets is 5 mg, 10 ÷ 5 = 2

EXERCISE NINE

1 13 500 mcg   3 mcg × 75 kg × 60 minutes

2 13.5 mg   13 500 ÷ 1000

3 324 mg or 0.324 g   13.5 × 24 hours

4 4.125 mg   2.5 mg × 1.65 m²

5 24.75 mg   4.125 mg × 6 doses

6 20 mg/ml   10 g = 10 000 mg ÷ 500 ml

7 15 ml   300 mg ÷ 20 mg/ml

8 0.9 grams   300 mg × 3 doses = 900 mg ÷ 1000

9 a & b, see fluid balance chart (Fig. 1.5)

10 9 December   2 March + 7 days + 9 months

11 See observation chart (Fig 1.6)

12 See observation chart (Fig 1.6)

13 3 in 5   300 in 500 becomes 3 in 5

14 **a** 1000 ml
    b 100 ml per hour   1000 ml ÷ 10 hours

15 300 ml

16 Yes, it is close enough

17 172–173 ml/hour   690 ml ÷ 4 hours

18 2.87 ml per minute   172 ml/hour ÷ 60 minutes

19 57 drops per minute   2.87 ml × 20 drops/ml

20 200 ml × 20 drops per $\dfrac{200}{2} \times \dfrac{20}{60}$
    ml ÷ 2 hours × 60 minutes

EXERCISE TEN

1	**a** 1/2	**b** 3/5	**c** 3/10	**d** 1/10
2	**a** 0.4	**b** 0.25	**c** 0.4	**d** 0.25
3	**a** 10%	**b** 30%	**c** 30%	**d** 15%
4	**a** 1 in 3	**b** 2 to 3	**c** 2 in 5	**d** 1 in 5
5	**a** 4 to 21	**b** 7 to 18	**c** 3 to 1	**d** 1 to 1

	Ward	
FLINDERS MEDICAL CENTRE	Surname	LEE
FLUID BALANCE	Other Names	Jenny Heather
CHART	D.O.B./Sex	30-11-1980 female
Medical Officer: *S. Jones*	Date: 14 . 2 . 2003	Address / Medi. No.	987 654 321

	INTAKE				OUTPUT				
Time	By Mouth or Tube (Description)	ml	Intravenous	ml	Vomitus or Aspirate	ml	Faeces and Other Drainage (Description)	ml	Urine ml
0100	Water (360)								
0200									
0300									
0400									
0500									
0600	Water (1000)	100							430
0700	Tea (150)	150							
0800									
0900									300
1000	Tea (150)	150							
1100					Vomitus	300			
1200	Soup (200)	200							
1300	Tea (150)	75							
1400	Water (1000)	1000							
1500	Tea (150)	150							
1600									
1700	Jelly (150)	150							150
1800	Tea (150)	75							
1900									
2000	Tea (150)	150			Vomitus	250			
2100									300
2200									
2300									
2400	Water	780							
Total		2980				550			1180
	Grand Total........	2980					Grand Total........	1730	

(Not Including Insensible Loss) 600
Total 2330
(Plus)
Balance 650
Minus

Total Volume of Blood Infused..

Figure 1.5

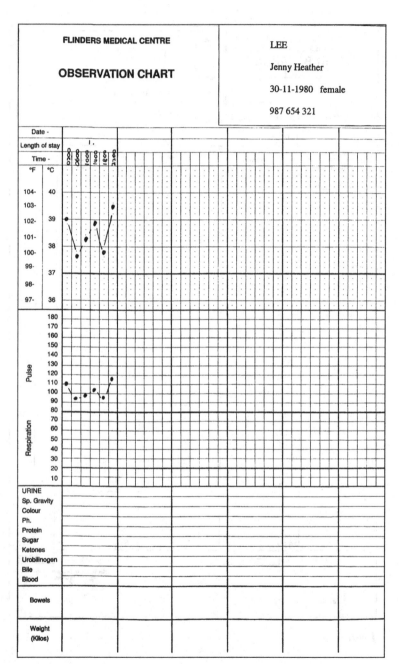

Figure 1.6

6 **a** 1 to 4   **b** 3 to 17   **c** 1 in 5   **d** 2 in 3

7 **a** 7 in 8   **b** 2 in 3   **c** 3 in 4   **d** 1 in 2

8 **a** 4 to 1   **b** 1 in 4   **c** 1 in 5   **d** 1 to 9

9 **a** 1 to 5   **b** 3 to 5   **c** 3 to 2   **d** 1 to 2

10 **a** 3 to 2   **b** 1 in 3   **c** 3 in 4   **d** 1 in 2

11 1 to 19

12 1 to 4

13 35%

14 800 ml

15 160 milk, 40 ml water

16 100 ml

17 40 ml of 6%, 20 ml of solvent
$$\frac{4}{100} \div \frac{6}{100} \times \frac{60}{1} =$$
$$\frac{4}{100} \times \frac{100}{6} \times \frac{60}{1}$$

18 9 grams
$$\frac{0.9}{100} = \frac{9}{1000} \times \frac{1000}{1}$$

19 50 grams
$$\frac{5}{100} \times \frac{1000}{1}$$

20 31 females to 7 males
$$\frac{35}{155} = \frac{7}{31}$$

2

Medications

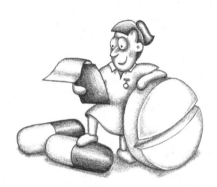

Objectives

After completing the given calculations, it is expected that you should be able to:

1 calculate basic mathematical sums including decimal and percentage calculations

2 demonstrate an understanding of the concept of ratios

3 calculate the dosages of oral medication, including mixtures

4 calculate the rate of flow in ml/hour and drops/minute for intravenous infusions and nasogastric feeds

5 calculate dosages for parenteral medications

EXERCISE ONE

ORAL MEDICATIONS—TABLETS

Oral medications are drugs that are given by mouth. In this exercise, we will consider only tablets or capsules. Sometimes tablets that you are required to give need to be broken. A tablet that has one or two indented marks is said to be 'scored' which allows the tablet to be broken smoothly.

 Example

single scored   double scored

Figure 2.1

A formula is generally used to calculate the correct dose of medication to be given. However, it is frequently obvious what the dose should be. For example, suppose the order is for 40 mg of a drug to be given and the tablets available are 20 mg per tablet—you do not need a formula to tell you to give two tablets!

It is very important that you check that the answer 'looks right'. For example, if, after working out your calculation you came up with the answer to give four or five tablets, *then you need to check that your calculation is correct!* In most cases, but not always, you would not give so many tablets from one order.

 Example

Mrs Jones has an order for paracetamol (Panamax), 1 gram, 'O', 4-hourly prn for pain.

- 'O' or 'po' means that this medication is to be given orally or by mouth.
- '4-hourly' (4/24) means that this medication can be, or is to be given every 4 hours.
- 'prn' or PRN means *pro re nata*; it is the Latin for 'as necessary' or whenever required by the client.

Panamax*

Paracetamol Tablets
Each TABLET contains PARACETAMOL 500 mg

sanofi~synthelabo   AUST R 15490   **100 Tablets**

This order indicates that Mrs Jones may have 1 g of paracetamol (Panamax) by mouth, every 4 hours if she has pain or feels that she needs this medication.

If the order is given in a different unit to that of the available stock (in this case 1 g is ordered, stock available is 500 mg), convert the order to the same unit, and convert 1 g to mg.

 Formula

$$\frac{\text{Strength required}}{\text{Strength available}} \text{ or } \frac{1000 \text{ mg}}{500 \text{ mg}} \text{ or } 1000 \div 500 = 2$$

a Jim Smith is to have 250 mcg of Lanoxin each day. Check the label on the package for the dosage per tablet and calculate the number of tablets he should be given each day.

PRESCRIPTION ONLY MEDICINE
KEEP OUT OF REACH OF CHILDREN

LANOXIN
250 micrograms
Digoxin Tablets
Each tablet contains
DIGOXIN 250 micrograms
100 TABLETS   SIGMA
AUST R 15333

b Jane Ellis is to have 25 mg of oral Pethidine twice a day. Check the label for the dosage and calculate the number of tablets she should be given per dose.

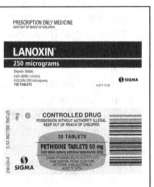

CONTROLLED DRUG
POSSESSION WITHOUT AUTHORITY ILLEGAL.
KEEP OUT OF REACH OF CHILDREN.

20 TABLETS
PETHIDINE TABLETS 50 mg
Each tablet contains pethidine hydrochloride 50mg
SIGMA PHARMACEUTICALS PTY LTD.
3408 CENTRE ROAD, CLAYTON,
VICTORIA 3169 AUSTRALIA
AUST R 10764

c Ron Cook is to have 45 mg of Pheno-barbitone each night. Check the dosage per tablet on the label and calculate the number of tablets he should be given each night.

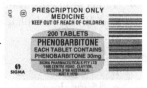

PRESCRIPTION ONLY
MEDICINE
KEEP OUT OF REACH OF CHILDREN
200 TABLETS
PHENOBARBITONE
EACH TABLET CONTAINS
PHENOBARBITONE 30mg
SIGMA PHARMACEUTICALS PTY LTD
1408 CENTRE ROAD, CLAYTON,
VICTORIA 3168 AUSTRALIA.
AUST R 18750
SIGMA

d Molly Wise is to have 250 mg of Amoxycillin & Clavulanic Acid every 6 hours. Check the label and state the number of tablets that should be given per dose.

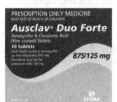

PRESCRIPTION ONLY MEDICINE
KEEP OUT OF REACH OF CHILDREN
Ausclav° Duo Forte
Amoxycillin & Clavulanic Acid
(film coated) Tablets
10 tablets
875/125 mg
SIGMA

Answers:
You should have given Jim Smith 1 tablet, Jane Ellis ½ a tablet, Ron Cook 1½ tablets and Molly Wise 2 tablets.

Activity

1 You have 500 mg tablets. Calculate the following number of tablets to be given
   a Order 250 mg
   b Order 750 mg
   c Order 1 g
   d Order 1.25 g

2 You are to give 100 mg of drug A. Calculate this dose from the following available stock
   a 50 mg/tablet
   b 200 mg/tablet
   c 25 mg/tablet
   d 100 mg/tablet

3 Stock strength available is equivalent to 0.25 g. Calculate the number of tablets required for a
   a 250 mg dose
   b 125 mg dose
   c 0.5 g dose
   d 750 mg dose

4 Tablet strengths available for drug B are 100 mg, 50 mg, 20 mg and 10 mg. Calculate which strength and how many tablets you should give for a
   a 75 mg dose
   b 80 mg dose
   c 15 mg dose
   d 150 mg dose

From the following stock strengths, calculate the number of tablets to be given

5 a Want 250 mg, have 1 g
   b Want 0.005 mg, have 5 mcg
   c Want 250 mg, have 0.5 g
   d Want 250 mg, have 0.25 g

6 a Want 1.5 g, have 750 mg
   b Want 0.005 mg, have 5 mcg
   c Want 0.001 mg, have 1 mcg
   d Want 150 mg, have 0.3 g

7 a Have 250 mg, want 0.25 g
   b Have 0.25 mg, want 250 mcg
   c Have 1 g, want 1500 mg
   d Have 62.5 mcg, want 0.125 mg

8 a Have 0.4 g, want 200 mg
   b Have 1.2 g, want 600 mg
   c Have 0.05 mg, want 25 mcg
   d Have 400 mg, want 0.6 g

9 a Want 25 mg, have 100 mg
   b Have 600 mcg, want 0.3 mg
   c Have 5 mg, want 10 mg
   d Want 150 mcg, have 0.05 mg

10 a Want 50 mcg, have 0.05 mg
    b Have 40 mg, want 0.08 g
    c Want 10 mg, have 0.01 g
    d Have 375 mg, want 0.75 g

11 Your client is ordered 250 mg of drug A. If stock available contains 500 mg of drug A in a scored tablet, how many tablets should you give to your client?

12 A man is ordered 500 mg of drug B. If stock available is equivalent to 0.25 g tablets, how many tablets should he be given?

13 A child is ordered 62.5 mcg of drug C. If stock on hand is double scored 0.25 mg tablets, what should the child be given?

14 A child is ordered 150 mg of drug D. If stock in the ward is equivalent to 0.3 g tablets, how many tablets should the child be given?

15 a Your client is ordered 1.5 g of drug E each day, to be given 8-hourly in three equally divided doses. Calculate the dose of each administration.

   b If stock available in the ward is 250 mg capsules, how many capsules should be given per dose?

16 a A child is ordered 100 mcg of drug F each day, to be given 6-hourly or in four equally divided doses. Calculate the amount of drug F that should be given per dose.

   b Drug F is available in double scored tablets with the equivalent value of 0.05 mg per tablet. What should this child be given?

17 a A man is ordered 2 g of drug G per day, to be given in four equally divided doses. How many mg should he receive per dose?

   b If this medication is available as 250 mg capsules, how many capsules should he be given per dose?

18 a A child weighing 24 kg is to have 10 mg of drug H per kilogram of body weight per day. Calculate a single dose of this medication if it is to be given 4-hourly.

   b Calculate the number of tablets to be given if the ward stocks 20 mg tablets.

19 a A woman with a body surface area of 1.5 m^2 is to have 2 g of drug J per m^2 of body surface area each day, to be given 4-hourly. Calculate a single dose of this medication.

b If stock available is 500 mg capsules, how many should she be given per dose?

20 a A man weighing 60 kg is to have 5 mg of drug K per kilogram of body weight each day, to be given 8-hourly. How many mg should he receive each dose?

b If stock in the ward consists of 100 mg tablets, how many tablets should he receive per dose?

EXERCISE TWO

ORAL MEDICATIONS—MIXTURES

Many people, especially children, find it difficult to swallow tablets, and for this reason drugs are often made up into a liquid format. For this exercise we will consider oral mixtures, syrups and elixirs. Syrups are mixtures which have sugar added and elixirs are drugs that have been mixed with an alcohol base because the drug does not readily dissolve in water.

Again, a formula is generally used to calculate the correct volume of mixture to be poured and given.

 Example

Sally is to have 150 mg of Amoxil syrup for her chest infection. Amoxil syrup is available at a strength or concentration of 125 mg of Amoxil in every 5 ml of syrup. Calculate the volume of medicine that will be needed for her.

 Formula

$$\frac{\text{Dose prescribed}}{\text{Stock strength}} \times \frac{\text{Volume in which stock strength is dissolved}}{1}$$

$$\frac{150}{125} \times \frac{5}{1} = \frac{750}{125} = 6 \text{ ml of syrup}$$

You should pour 6 ml of Amoxil syrup for Sally.

Activity

Calculate the volume of medicine to be poured for each of the following exercises.

1 a Want 150 mg, have 25 mg/ml
   b Want 40 mg, have 10 mg/ml
   c Want 0.1 g, have 20 mg/ml
   d Want 50 mg, have 10 mg/ml
   e Want 25 mg, have 5 mg/ml
   f Want 200 mg, have 25 mg/ml
   g Want 0.5 g, have 125 mg/2 ml
   h Want 60 mg, have 20 mg/ml
2 a Want 0.2 g, have 20 mg/2 ml
   b Want 60 mg, have 3 g/100 ml
   c Want 0.25 g, have 1 g/100 ml
   d Want 40 mg, have 5 mg/ml
   e Want 240 mg, have 120 mg/2 ml
   f Want 75 mg, have 5 g/500 ml
   g Want 125 mcg, have 25 mcg/ml
   h Want 0.5 g, have 100 mg/5 ml
3 a Want 0.9 mg, have 150 mcg/2 ml
   b Want 0.5 g, have 125 mg/2 ml
   c Want 0.6 g, have 150 mg/2 ml
   d Want 45 mg, have 15 mg/ml
   e Want 1.5 g, have 500 mg/5 ml
   f Want 600 mg, have 100 mg/ml
   g Want 450 mg, have 0.05 g/ml
   h Want 0.1 g, have 1 g/10 ml
4 a Want 25 mg, have 0.01 g/ml
   b Want 60 mg, have 50 mg/ml
   c Want 750 mg, have 250 mg/ml
   d Want 75 mg, have 15 mg/ml
   e Want 750 mg, have 125 mg/2 ml
   f Want 80 mg, have 40 mg/ml
   g Want 500 mg, have 100 mg/ml
   h Want 250 mg, have 1 g/4 ml

When giving a medication in the liquid format, it is important to note that medications are sometimes ordered by volume (in ml rather than mg) and it is your responsibility to ensure that the dose that you give is within the normal limits for that client.

Example

Emma, who is six years old, has been ordered 6 ml of paracetamol (Panadol) for her earache. You are aware that the paracetamol comes in two strengths: 24 mg/ml and 48 mg/ml. Both strengths are available in the ward drug trolley, so how do you know which one to use? It is **your responsibility to check** which medication is suitable for Emma. Too much of the drug is undesirable (and could be dangerous), and too little would be ineffective.

On checking the 'MIMS' (2001, 4-416), the drug information book available in the ward, you note that children should receive 15 mg of paracetamol (Panadol) per kg of body weight per dose. Emma is 20 kg. Thus, 20 kg × 15 mg/kg = 300 mg. Next, find the appropriate dose (in mg) for the ordered volume.

Formula

$$\frac{\text{Volume ordered}}{\text{Volume available}} \times \frac{\text{Dose contained in volume available}}{1}$$

Let us consider, now, both of the medications that are available in the drug trolley.

$$\frac{6\ \text{ml}}{1\ \text{ml}} \times \frac{24\ \text{mg}}{1} = 144\ \text{mg} \quad \text{or} \quad \frac{6\ \text{ml}}{1\ \text{ml}} \times \frac{48\ \text{mg}}{1} = 288\ \text{mg}$$

Emma should have the strength of 48 mg/ml for this medication to be effective.

Activity

5 a Scott is to have 10 ml of drug A. Stock available is 125 mg/5 ml. How much medication (drug A) is Scott having per dose?

b If Scott weighs 10 kg and the normal dose of this medication is 25 mg/kg of body weight, is this dose within normal limits?

6 a Sharon is to have 8 ml of drug B. Stock available is 250 mg/ 5 ml. What is the actual dose of this medication that Sharon will receive?

  b Sharon, who has a body surface area of 0.8 m², is permitted 500 mg of drug B per m² of body surface area per dose. Is the ordered dose within normal limits?

7 a Peter is to have 12 ml of drug C. Stock available is a 100 ml bottle containing 2 g of drug C. What dose of drug C will Peter receive from this order?

  b Peter's weight is 20 kg and it is recommended that the dose he receives should be 12.5 mg/kg of body weight per day. Is the ordered dose within normal limits for Peter?

8 a Sara is to have 6 ml of drug D. Stock available is a 0.5 L bottle containing 5 grams of drug D. How many mg of drug D is in a 6 ml dose?

  b Sara, who has a body surface area of 0.6 m², is permitted 100 mg of drug D per m² of body surface area. Is her dose within acceptable limits?

Six-year-old James has been admitted to hospital with a severe chest infection. He weighs 20 kg and has a body surface area of 0.8 m². James is pyretic, has a productive cough and is very fretful.

9 James is to have 40 mg of Amoxil (an antibiotic to fight the infection) per kilogram of body weight per day. How much Amoxil per day should he receive?

10 The above medication is to be given 6/24 (6-hourly). Calculate the dose, in mg, for a single administration of this medication.

11 What volume of medication should be poured if the available stock has a concentration of 125 mg/5 ml?

12 When you take James's temperature you notify the registered nurse that it is 40.2°C. 10 ml of paracetamol (Panadol) elixir is ordered and this mixture has a concentration of 120 mg/5 ml. How many mg of paracetamol will he receive?

13 According to the 'MIMS', James is permitted 15 mg/kg of body weight/dose. Is the ordered dose within these limits?

14 James is to drink more fluid. You are to encourage him to drink 100 ml of fluid every half hour for the next 8 hours. How much fluid will be charted for this period if you are successful in persuading him to drink this amount?

15 James asks for some weak apple juice. How much juice would be required to make him a 200 ml glass of juice at a 4 to 1 ratio?

16 Later in the day James develops a rash. It is suspected that he has an allergy to Amoxil, which is then ceased. He is to be given 12.5 mg of an antihistamine, Phenergan, to treat the rash. This medication is available as a mixture with a concentration of 5 mg/5 ml. How much should you pour for him?

17 Another antibiotic, Bactrim, is commenced. James is to have 120 mg of Bactrim per m^2 of body surface area per day. What is his daily dose of this medication?

18 How many mg would be in a single dose if this medication is to be given BD (twice daily)?

19 What volume of this medication should you pour if the stock available has a concentration of 40 mg/5 ml?

James continues to be fretful and is refusing to drink the fluids offered to him. An intravenous infusion is established and James is to have 300 ml over the next two hours and the remainder of fluid over a seven-hour period.

20 a How many ml per hour should he receive from the order for 300 ml over 2 hours?

    b What volume per hour should be delivered for the remainder of the 1 L of fluid?

EXERCISE THREE

Activity
Complete the following computations

1 a Jack is ordered 8 ml of paracetamol and stock available is 120 mg/5 ml. How many mg of paracetamol will Jack receive per dose?

b Mary is to have 144 mg of paracetamol and the available stock contains 120 mg/5 ml. What volume of medication should be poured to fulfil this order?

c Tom has been ordered 375 mg of drug A and stock on hand is 0.25 g scored tablets. How many tablets should he be given?

d Chris is to have 0.4 mg of drug B. If the available stock is 200 mcg tablets, how many tablets should he be given?

e James has been ordered 0.2 g of drug C. This medication is available as a mixture with a concentration of 125 mg/5 ml. What volume should be poured for him?

f An elderly lady, who is having difficulty swallowing tablets, has been ordered drug D, 750 mg. This medication is available as a mixture, 0.25 g/5 ml. What volume should you pour?

g Aspirin 0.6 g has been ordered for a young man. This medication is available as a mixture, 150 mg/5 ml. What volume should be poured to fulfil this order?

h 25 mg of drug E has been ordered. If available stock is 12.5 mg tablets, how many tablets should this man receive?

i 450 mg of drug F has been ordered. Stock on hand is 0.3 g scored tablets. How many tablets should this man be given?

j 375 mg of drug G has been ordered. The only stock on hand is 125 mg tablets. How many tablets should be given?

Activity

Your employment in the nursing home is continuing and today one of your clients is an elderly lady called Mrs Rose Emmett. She is receiving respite care while her daughter is having a holiday. You note that her nursing notes state that she is 5 feet 3 inches tall and that she weighs 7 stone.

2 **a** Remembering that there are 12 inches in 1 foot and that 2.54 cm equals 1 inch, convert her height to cm.

   b Taking into account that there are 14 pounds in every stone and that 2.2 pounds equals 1 kg, convert her weight to kg.

The registered nurse asks you if you would like to observe her doing this lady's medications so that you have an idea of the principles involved in this task.

3   **a** Mrs Emmett has 1.5 g of drug A each day, given in three equally divided doses. How many mg would she have in a single dose?

    b If each tablet has 500 mg, how many tablets should she receive per dose?

4 She has a heart tablet twice a day. If each tablet contains 250 mcg, what is her daily dose in mg?

5   **a** Her bottle of cough mixture contains 200 ml of medicine. If she has 20 ml of mixture twice a day, how long should the bottle last?

    b If each ml of fluid in this bottle contains 0.001 mg of drug B, how many mcg of drug B does the bottle contain?

Mrs Emmett, who is quite frail, has been commenced on nasogastric tube feeds. She is to have an 8-ounce bottle of Osmolite every 3 hours from 06.00 to 21.00. You are aware that 8 ounces of fluid is equal to 237 ml.

6   **a** What is her daily total fluid volume, in ml, from the tube feeds?

    b If each feed is followed by 60 ml of water to flush the tubing, how much water would be added to her fluid balance chart for the day?

7 If every ml of this lady's tube feed is made up of 14 drops as it passes through the transparent drip chamber, how many potential drops are there in her 237 ml feed?

8 Taking into account that this feed is to last for 60 minutes, how many drops per minute will pass through the transparent chamber?

9 Remembering that the 237 ml is to last for 60 minutes, how many ml per minute should she receive?

10 Having calculated the number of drops per minute, and bearing in mind that 14 drops make one ml, do your answers for Q 8 and 9 match?

Later that day, Mrs Emmett complains of feeling nauseated and tells you she thinks she will be sick. A decision is made to drip her 18.00 feed at 28 drops per minute.

11 a Remembering that 14 drops make up one ml, how many ml of
fluid is she receiving every minute from this new order?

b How long would you expect this 237 ml bottle of feed to last?

12 She is offered a medication to help reduce her nausea. The
mixture contains 2 mg per ml and she is to have 10 mg. How
much medicine would you expect to be poured?

When you next return to the nursing home, Mrs Emmett looks considerably better. Her nasogastric tube has been removed and she is
managing to eat a light, soft diet. You have been asked to encourage
her to drink more fluid.

13 Mrs Emmett asks you to make up a jug of lime cordial for her.
Instructions on the bottle indicate that a 10% solute is required to reconstitute the drink. How much cordial (solute) is required to make up a 200 ml glass of drink?

14 a How much iced water is required to complete this task?

b What is the ratio of cordial to water (V/V)?

c Write the solute as a decimal.

Mrs Emmett has a small ulcer on her foot and you are observing the
registered nurse as she prepares to clean and redress the ulcer. Before
she gets the equipment, she asks Mrs Emmett if she would like any-
thing for the pain caused by the dressing procedure. She says she
would like the usual tablets.

15 She is permitted 1 g of drug C and the tablets available are 500 mg
ones. How many tablets would you expect her to be given?

16 The solution for cleaning the ulcer needs to be diluted because it
stings the raw surface area of the wound. From the 0.9% stock
available, a 0.3% solution is to be made up. How much 0.9%
solution is required to make up 60 ml of 0.3%?

17 How much sterile water will be required to complete the task?

18 At 18.00, her medications are due again. Her heart tablets have
been reduced to 125 mcg per dose. Stock tablets are equivalent to
0.25 mg, so what should she be given?

19 She is ordered 10 ml of mixture for her constipation. If each ml of mixture contains 25 mg of medication D, how many mg will she receive per dose?

20 As Mrs Emmett was being settled for the night, her sleeping tablets were brought to her. She needed 7.5 mg of drug E and the available stock was 5 mg available tablets. How many tablets would you expect her to be given?

EXERCISE FOUR

Activity

You are assisting the registered nurse with the morning washes in a six-bed bay in a hospital ward. The nurse in charge of the ward is very conscious of the costs involved in running the ward and has strategically placed a notice informing staff of laundry costs.

Item	Price	Item	Price
Quilts	$1.439	Gowns	$0.596
Blankets	1.832	Bath towels	0.373
Sheets	1.063	Face cloths	0.04
Draw sheets	0.80	Baby gowns	0.099
Pillow cases	0.197	Baby vests	0.032
Pyjamas	1.064	Napkins	0.103

1 Mrs Cottee, with a chest infection, has spilt her breakfast and requires a top sheet and pillow case. She would also like a clean towel and face cloth. What is the cost of her fresh linen?

2 Mrs Rayner is still very unsteady following a fall at home and has knocked over her washbowl. She needs a clean quilt, blanket, two sheets and two pillow cases. How much will all this cost?

3 Miss Stanley, who is recovering from a stroke, has wet her bed. She requires two sheets, a draw sheet and a pillow case. What is the cost for her clean linen?

4 Jane Rix is going home today and so all her linen (quilt, blanket, two sheets, two pillow cases, one towel and a face cloth) will need replacing. How much will this cost?

5 Patty Dawson is now up and about and so has showered herself and made her own bed but would like a clean towel and face cloth. What will this cost?

6 Mrs Jolson has her three-week-old baby as a boarder. Mrs Jolson has a fever and her sheets are wet with perspiration. She needs a pillow case, two sheets, a clean towel and a face cloth. Her baby needs a vest, gown and nappy, what is the total cost for mother and baby?

7 What is the total cost of laundry for this bay?

8 If the cost of this six-bed bay is approximately equal to all other bays in this ward, what would be the cost for a 30-bed ward?

9 This hospital has 800 beds. What could one expect the average morning linen change to cost?

10 How much would this be for one year?

You are interested in some of the statistics about women's health which are also displayed in the ward.

11 Each year, approximately 1000 women are diagnosed with cervical cancer and 350 women die from the disease. What percentage of women survive this condition?

12 In one state of Australia 63 542 women gave birth to an infant during the year, 86% of the women were under the age of 34 years. How many women were over the age of 34 years?

13 Only 4.3% of the births were to women under the age of 20 years. How many is this?

14 40.7% of all women who gave birth in this year had a spontaneous labour and birth. How many women needed some form of intervention to assist with the birth process?

15 A follow-up study indicated that 14.6% of the women studied during that year suffered postnatal depression following the birth of the infant. How many women would this be?

After morning tea, at 10.00, you are invited to observe the registered nurse doing a medication round. She requests that you attempt to work out all the calculations involved in this task.

16 **a** Mrs Cottee is to have 750 mg of drug A, three times per day. Write a single dose in grams.

b What is the total daily dose (in grams) of this medication for Mrs Cottee?

c If this medication is available in 500 mg tablets, what should she be given for this 14.00 dose?

17 **a** Mrs Rayner's intravenous infusion can be removed when the present bag of fluid completes, and 180 ml remains in the bag. If each ml equals 20 drops, how many potential drops are in the bag?

b It is currently dripping at 30 drops per minute. Remembering the number of drops that make one ml, how many ml is she receiving every hour?

c How long (in hours) would you expect this bag to last?

18 **a** Miss Stanley is to have 8 ml of medicine containing 40 mg of drug B. How many mg of drug B are there in one ml of this medicine?

b How long could you expect the 200 ml bottle to last if she is to have this medicine every 6 hours?

Mrs Jolson is to have an intravenous antibiotic, 600 mg every 8 hours. This medication is available as 1 gram of powder and is to be mixed with sterile water to form an injectable solution.

19 **a** If the concentration of this medicated powder is to be 100 mg per ml, how much fluid (solution) would you expect to be in the bottle when the water and powder mix?

b How many ml of fluid would you expect the nurse to draw up for the 600 mg dose?

20 **a** Patty Dawson is to have 0.25 mg of drug C. Write this dose in mcg.

b The only tablets available are 125 mcg per tablet, therefore how many tablets would you expect this lady to receive?

Having completed the exercises in relation to oral medications, go to the website (see p. x) to establish just how much knowledge you have acquired to date. Try to complete the quizzes in Module Two, Assessments One and Two in 20 minutes each.

EXERCISE FIVE

INTRAVENOUS FLUID MANAGEMENT

If people are unable to tolerate food or fluids by mouth, or if there is a need to give extra fluids, an intravenous infusion could be established. In this situation, specially prepared sterile fluid is introduced directly into the circulatory system via a vein.

When an intravenous line is established, it usually consists of a bag of fluid suspended from an intravenous pole, connected to a thin plastic tube, which delivers the fluid (via a plastic cannula which is positioned in the person's vein), directly into the circulatory system.

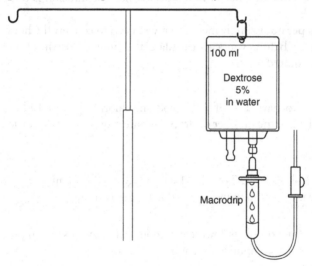

Figure 2.2 *Intravenous line*

When fluid is given intravenously, a formula may be used to work out how fast you will need to drip the fluid to give the required amount over the specified period of time. **The most commonly used drop factor for intravenous giving sets in Australia is 20 drops per ml, referred to as the drop factor (D/F).** The giving set is called a *macro* set and is used mostly for adults. A *micro* giving set emits 60 drops per ml and is used for children. There are infusion lines with alternative drop factors, for example a giving set which emits 15 drops per ml is still in use in some Australian states when blood is being administered.

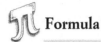

Formula

$$\frac{\text{Volume ml}}{\text{Time (hours)}} \times \frac{\text{Drop factor (drops/ml)}}{\text{Minutes (60 minutes/hour)}} = \text{Drops/Minute}$$

- The **volume** is the amount of fluid that has been ordered by the medical practitioner.
- The **drop factor** is the number of drops leaving the drip chamber that make up 1 ml of fluid and this will depend on the size of the outlet within the drip chamber.
- The **time** is the number of hours over which the infusion is to be delivered.
- **Minutes per hour** simply means that you need to convert the hours to minutes before you can calculate the number of drops per minute required.

Example

Mr Smith is to have 1 L of 0.9% sodium chloride over a 10-hour period. Calculate the number of drops/minute required for this order.

Formula

$$\frac{\text{Vol}}{\text{Time}} \times \frac{\text{D/F}}{60 \text{ mins}} \quad \text{or} \quad \frac{1000 \text{ ml}}{10 \text{ hrs}} \times \frac{20 \text{ drops/ml}}{60 \text{ minutes}}$$

Reduce the fraction to its lowest common denominators to simplify the mathematical computation required.
For example:

$$\frac{1000}{10} \times \frac{20}{60} = \frac{100}{3} \text{ or } 33.33 \text{ drops/minute}$$

Mr Smith's solution should infuse at the rate of 33 drops/minute.

What you have actually done is to find the number of potential drops in the bag of fluid (1000 ml × 20 drops/ml) and divided this figure by the number of minutes (10 hours × 60 minutes/hour) over which the infusion has been ordered to run.

This principle is the same regardless of the volume, time or drop factor.

Once you have calculated the number of drops that are to be delivered each minute, you need to be able to work out how this will be done. Should you be observing a registered nurse carrying out this task, it may appear to you that this is a very simple exercise, and it is, once you become proficient at it! So, let us begin.

Your answer above is 33 drops per minute. Make the task easier by trying to regulate the number of drops over a quarter of a minute. How many drops would you expect to see leaving the drip chamber every 15 seconds for the above scenario? 33 ÷ 4 = 8.25, approximately 8 every 15 seconds or one drop in almost two seconds. Next:

- Check that the roller clamp (which regulates the flow rate) is close to the drip chamber so that both are readily visible to you.
- Position yourself so that the chamber is at eye level.
- Hold your watch close to the chamber so that the watch and chamber are both visible to you.
- Adjust the roller clamp (either up or down) until approximately 8 drops fall every 15 seconds.
- Check the drops per minute for a full minute and adjust again as required.

Sometimes an intravenous line will contain a burette, or a volume control device, and in this case you will be required to calculate the volume of fluid that is to run into this device every hour. This task is quite simple: simply divide the volume (in ml) by the number of ordered hours.

Example

Mr Smith is to have 1 L over a 10-hour period. Calculate the number of ml/hr to be given.

Formula

$$\frac{\text{Volume (ml)}}{\text{Time (hours)}} \text{ or } \frac{1000}{10} = 100 \text{ ml/hour}$$

Mr Smith should receive 100 ml every hour for this order.

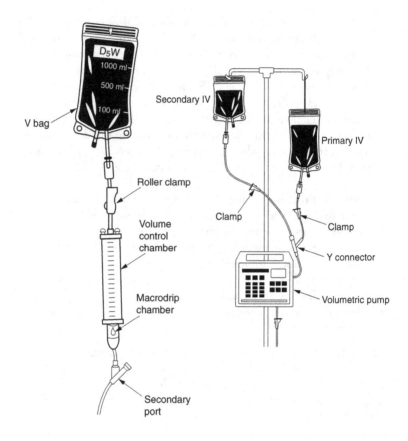

Figure 2.3 *Burette*   **Figure 2.4** *Volumetric pump*

Activity

1 **a** 600 ml is to be infused over a 4-hour period. The drop factor
        (D/F) for the giving set is 20 drops per ml. Calculate the
        volume per hour and the number of drops per minute (dpm)
        that are required for this order.
   b 500 ml is to infuse over a 5-hour period. The drop factor for
        this giving set is 15 drops/ml. Calculate the volume per hour
        and the number of drops per minute that are required for this
        order.

c 1200 ml has been ordered to infuse over a 6-hour period. The drop factor for this giving set is 20 drops per ml. Calculate the volume per hour and the number of drops per minute that are required for this order.

2 Calculate the volume per hour required for the following orders
  a 400 ml over 5 hours   **b** 150 ml over 2 hours
  c 200 ml over 2 hours   **d** 750 ml over 3 hours
  e 450 ml over 3 hours   **f** 300 ml over 6 hours

3 Calculate the drops per minute required to deliver the following orders if the drop factor for the giving set is 60 drops per ml
  a 1000 ml over 16 hours   **b** 500 ml over 10 hours
  c 340 ml over 4 hours   **d** 800 ml over 10 hours
  e 350 ml over 7 hours   **f** 100 ml over 1 hour

4 Calculate the drops per minute required to deliver the following orders if the drop factor for the giving set is 20 drops per ml

  a 750 ml over 5 hours   **b** 600 ml over 4 hours
  c 500 ml over 3 hours   **d** 1000 ml over 10 hours
  e 900 ml over 6 hours   **f** 150 ml over 1 hour

5 Calculate the rates of flow (in drops/minute) for blood transfusions if the drop factor for the giving set is 15 drops/ml

  a 300 ml over 3 hours   **b** 150 ml over 1 hour
  c 350 ml over 2 hours   **d** 600 ml over 8 hours
  e 450 ml over 4 hours   **f** 0.4 L over 5 hours

Stop now and consider the role played by drop factors. While in Australia the drop factors may remain consistent, it is important that you understand that different countries may have different giving sets with different drop factors. The difference in the size of the outlet, which controls the size of the drop, greatly influences the rate of flow, or the number of drops actually delivering the ordered volume. Take note of this in the following exercises.

6 In the following exercises, 1000 ml is to infuse over a 10-hour period. Using the different drop factors for each example, calculate the rates of flow in drops per minute

a the drop factor is 10   b the drop factor is 12
c the drop factor is 14   d the drop factor is 15
e the drop factor is 20   f the drop factor is 60

Sometimes you are required to deliver a volume of fluid over a period of time that is less than one hour. In this case, you would still need to find the number of potential drops and then just simply divide this figure by the number of minutes over which the fluid ordered is to be delivered.

 ## Example

Tom Jones is to have 8 ml of his intravenous antibiotic added to the 22 ml of 5% dextrose currently in the burette of his infusion line, and infused over a 15-minute period. The drop factor (D/F) for the giving set is 20 drops/ml.

 ## Formula

$$\frac{22 + 8 \times 20}{15} \text{ or } \frac{30 \times 20}{15} = \frac{40}{1} \text{ or 40 drops/minute}$$

7 Calculate the following (in drops/minute) if the drop factor (D/F) is 20

a 50 ml over 20 minutes   b 100 ml over 40 minutes
c 45 ml over 15 minutes   d 40 ml over 10 minutes
e 20 ml over 15 minutes   f 60 ml over 12 minutes

8 Calculate the following (in drops/minute) if the drop factor (D/F) is 15

a 45 ml in 15 minutes   b 100 ml in 30 minutes
c 90 ml over 45 minutes   d 80 ml in 20 minutes
e 25 ml in 15 minutes   f 30 ml over 10 minutes

9 Calculate the following (in drops/minute) if the drop factor (D/F) is 60

    a 15 ml in 15 minutes   **b** 30 ml in 40 minutes
    c 45 ml in 60 minutes   **d** 20 ml in 20 minutes
    e 40 ml in 60 minutes   **f** 20 ml in 40 minutes

10 Calculate the following

    a 30 ml/15 minutes, D/F 15   **b** 90 ml/45 minutes, D/F 15
    c 30 ml/45 minutes, D/F 60   **d** 60 ml/30 minutes, D/F 20
    e 45 ml/15 minutes, D/F 15   **f** 200 ml/60 minutes, D/F 14

It is also important to be able to calculate the time a given infusion, which is already in progress, will last. For example, Mr Black has an intravenous infusion in progress, and 120 ml remain in the bag. The drop factor for the giving set is 20 drops/ml and the infusion is dripping at 50 drops per minute. Mr Jones has been told he can go home when this infusion completes, and he asks you to give him a time for his wife to call to collect him.

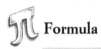 **Formula**

$$\frac{\text{Volume} \times \text{Drop factor}}{\text{Drops per minute}} \text{ or } \frac{120 \times 20}{50} = 48 \text{ minutes}$$

His wife can collect him in approximately 50 minutes time.

11 Using the given information, calculate the time that the following infusions will take to complete if the drop factor is 20
    a 150 ml, rate of flow 60 drops/min
    b 200 ml, rate of flow, 50 drops/min
    c 240 ml, rate of flow, 56 drops/min
    d 110 ml, rate of flow, 42 drops/min

12 Calculate the time of completion for the following infusions if the drop factor is 15
    a 180 ml, rate of flow 45 drops/min
    b 120 ml, rate of flow 30 drops/min
    c 120 ml, rate of flow 60 drops/min
    d 90 ml, rate of flow 30 drops/min

There are times when the client that you are caring for could have two lines in place. The main line has an attachment which is called a secondary or 'piggy back' line, and often this secondary line is used to deliver a medication. When two lines are in place, it is important to take into account the fluid from both lines when charting the client's intake on the fluid balance chart.

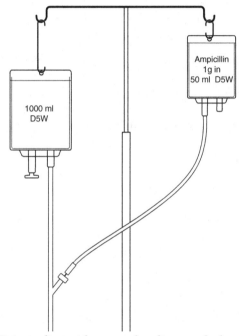

Figure 2.5 *Primary line with a secondary line attached*

Activity

13 Write the hourly volume of fluid that is being delivered for the following lines when both lines are in use

    a Main line 1 L over 8 hours, secondary line 100 ml over 2 hours

    b Main line 1 L over 10 hours, secondary line 100 ml over 10 hours

    c Main line 0.5 L over 6 hours, secondary line 50 ml over 60 minutes

    d Main line 1 L over 6 hours, secondary line 100 ml over 4 hours

Another aspect of intravenous infusion management is the ability to calculate the volume per minute or hour that is being administered. This is quite simple: just divide the number of drops per minute by the number of drops per ml that the giving set emits to get the ml/minute and then multiply by 60 to convert from ml/min to ml/hour.

 ## Example

Mr Peterson has been admitted to hospital for management of a heart condition. Because his heart is performing poorly, his medication orders state that he is to have no more than 30 ml of intravenous fluid per hour. A micro infusion set (60 drops/ml) is in place. This rate of flow in drops/min should be:

$$30 \text{ ml per hour} \quad \text{or} \quad \frac{30 \text{ ml} \times 60 \text{ drops/ml}}{60 \text{ minutes}} \quad \text{or} \quad 30 \text{ drops/minute}$$

When you check his infusion later in the day, it is dripping at the rate of 45 drops/minute. How much extra fluid is he having?

 ## Formula

$$\frac{\text{Drops per minute}}{\text{Drops per ml}} \quad \text{or} \quad \frac{45 \text{ drops/minute}}{60 \text{ drops/ml}} = 0.75 \text{ ml/min}$$

Mr Peterson is having 0.75 ml/min × 60 minutes rather than 0.5 ml × 60 minutes ordered. He is having 0.25 ml per minute extra, which is 15 ml/hour more than he is ordered.

14   Calculate the volume per minute for the following infusions if the drop factor is 20 drops/ml
   a 60 drops/minute   **b** 40 drops/minute
   c 10 drops/minute   **d** 20 drops/minute
   e 15 drops/minute   **f** 50 drops/minute

15   Calculate the volume per minute for the following infusions if the drop factor is 60 drops/ml
   a 30 drops/minute   **b** 20 drops/minute
   c 15 drops/minute   **d** 45 drops/minute
   e 60 drops/minute   **f** 75 drops/minute

16 Calculate the **ml/hour** for the following
   a 40 drops/minute, D/F 20   b 30 drops/minute, D/F 15
   c 45 drops/minute, D/F 60   d 50 drops/minute, D/F 20
   e 60 drops/minute, D/F 15   f 30 drops/minute, D/F 60

17 A client is to have 0.5 L of intravenous infusion over 4 hours. The drop factor for this giving set is 20 drops/ml. A secondary line is attached with 100 ml to be given over 5 hours. The drop factor for this line is 60 drops/ml. Calculate
   a the ml/hour and drops/minute for the main line
   b the drops/minute for the secondary line

18 Calculate
   a the total volume for both infusions over the first hour
   b the volume per hour for the main line only, if the rate of flow is increased to 50 drops/minute in the third hour
   c the time for completion of the secondary line if 40 ml remain in the bag and this line is dripping at the rate of 20 drops/minute

NASOGASTRIC TUBE FEEDS

Another way that fluid can be introduced into the body is via the gastro-intestinal system using a fine plastic catheter or tube if a person is unable to swallow safely. When this occurs, the nasogastric tube is inserted via the nose, into the stomach or the duodenum. One system that is in use for this purpose is the Osmolite tube feeding apparatus. Osmolite is the brand name for a specially prepared mixture with its own giving set, and feeds are available in bottles or cans, in 237 ml (or 8 fluid ounces) bottles and 946 ml dispensing cans.

   If these feeds are to be delivered over a specified period of time, then, as with the intravenous apparatus, a formula is used to regulate the rate of flow. This formula is the same as the one used for the intravenous infusion. The main difference being that the drop factor is 14 (which means that the drops are bigger and therefore less are required to make one ml) because Osmolite is thicker than intravenous fluid.

19 Using the formula given for intravenous fluids, calculate the rates of flow (in drops/minute) for nasogastric tube feeds if the drop factor for the giving set is 14 drops/ml

a 300 ml over 2 hours   b 1000 ml over 10 hours
c 350 ml over 1.5 hours   d 1800 ml over 20 hours
e 600 ml over 12 hours   f 250 ml over 1.5 hours

20 The solution to be delivered is Osmolite, via a nasogastric tube which has a drop factor of 14. Calculate the following in drops/minute

a 2.5 L over 20 hours   b 1.5 L over 20 hours
c 1 L over 20 hours   d 300 ml over 1 hour
e 250 ml over 40 minutes   f 200 ml over 30 minutes

EXERCISE SIX

Activity

Complete the following computations

1 a Mary is ordered 10 ml of paracetamol and stock available is 120 mg/5 ml. How many mg of paracetamol will Mary receive for each dose?

b John is to have 160 mg of paracetamol and the available stock contains 120 mg/5 ml. What volume of medication should be poured to fulfil this order?

c Sarah has been ordered 125 mg of drug A and stock on hand is 0.25 g scored tablets. How many tablets should she be given?

d Jane is to have 0.2 mg of drug B. If the available stock is 200 mcg tablets, how many tablets should she be given?

e Peter has been ordered 0.25 g of drug C. This medication is available as a mixture with a concentration of 125 mg/5 ml, therefore what volume should be poured for him?

f An elderly man, who is having difficulty swallowing tablets, has been ordered 0.5 g of drug D. This medication is available as a mixture, 250 mg/5 ml. What volume should you pour?

g Aspirin 0.45 g has been ordered for a young man. This medication is available as a mixture, 50 mg/ml. What volume should be poured to fulfil this order?

h 25 mg of drug E has been ordered. Stock of this medication is 12.5 mg tablets, so how many tablets should this man receive?

    i 300 mg of drug F has been ordered. Stock on hand is 0.2 g scored tablets. How many tablets should this man be given?

    j 0.25 mg of drug G has been ordered. If stock on hand is 125 mcg tablets, how many tablets should be given?

You are on a clinical placement in a nursing home and you are observing the registered nurse doing a medication round. She asks you to calculate the number of tablets and the volume of any medications that need to be poured.

Mrs Sampson has high blood pressure, a mild heart condition, and a small but painful leg ulcer that needs to be attended to.

2   She is ordered 20 mg of frusemide (Lasix), a medication to assist in the removal of fluid from her body, each morning. If stock available is 40 mg scored tablets, how many tablets should she be given?

3   She has Lanoxin tablets for her weak heart and the dose is 125 mcg. Stock available is equivalent to 0.0625 mg tablets. How many tablets should she be given?

4   Capoten has been ordered for her high blood pressure. She has just been commenced on 10 mg BD. Stock available is an oral solution with a concentration of 5 mg/ml. What volume should be poured for her?

5   The Capoten mixture is to be diluted at a 1 in 50 (V/V) ratio. How much orange juice is required to achieve this ratio?

6   Mrs Sampson asks for 2 paracetamol (Panadol) for the pain in her leg. She is permitted 1 gram of this medication 4 hourly, PRN. If each tablet is 500 mg, and her last dose was yesterday evening, is this dose within her ordered limit?

7   Each day her leg ulcer is cleaned with 100 ml of 0.9% sodium chloride. How much actual sodium (salt) is there in this solution?

Mr Ryburn has had a cerebrovascular accident. At present he is receiving his nutrients via nasogastric tube feeds. His wife tells you that he weighs 12 stone 8 pounds, and his height is 6 feet 2 inches. His current nutritional intake is 25 calories/kg of body weight and he is being fed the commercial preparation called Osmolite.

8 Remembering that there are 14 pounds in each stone and 2.2 pounds in each kilogram, convert his weight to kilograms.

9 Remembering that there are 12 inches in each foot and 2.54 cm to each inch, convert his height to centimetres.

10 Taking into account that each calorie equals approximately 4 kilojoules, how many kilojoules should he be given each day?

11 Each bottle of Osmolite contains 237 ml and is followed by 20 ml of water to flush out the tube. If he is having eight feeds per day, what volume of fluid will be charted on the intake column of his fluid balance chart over a 24-hour period?

12 When each feed of 237 ml of Osmolite is being administered, it has potentially 14 drops per ml of fluid. How many potential drops would there be in one feed?

13 How many drops would need to drip each minute if this feed is to complete in 60 minutes?

Mrs Jenner is an elderly woman who is in the nursing home for respite care while her daughter has a holiday. She has developed a chest infection which is being treated with antibiotics.

14 She is to have 1 gram of Abbocillin each day, to be given in four equally divided doses. How many mg/dose should she receive?

15 This medication is available as 0.25 g capsules, so how many capsules should she be given/dose?

16 Mrs Jenner asks for something for her headache. She has an order for 750 mg of paracetamol (Panadol). Stock available is 0.5 g scored tablets, so what should she be given?

17 She is to have a cough expectorant to help her to cough up respiratory secretions. She is to have 10 ml of 'Bronchitis Mixture' every four hours. If each 10 ml of this mixture contains 110 mg of ammonium chloride, how much ammonium chloride will she have each day?

18 Following her midday meal, Mrs Jenner calls you and says she feels sick. She is ordered metoclopramide (Maxolon) tablets, 10 mg. Stock available is equivalent to 0.01 g. How many tablets should she be given?

19 Later, she asks for some 'weak apple juice'. You are to make up 200 ml of diluted apple juice at a 4 to 1 ratio of juice to water. How much ice water will you need to add to complete this task?

20 What percentage of this drink is water?

EXERCISE SEVEN

Activity

You are caring for a frail, elderly woman suffering from malnutrition and leg ulcers. She receives her nutrients via nasogastric tube feeds but can swallow sips of fluid and likes to suck sweets.

1 Prior to dressing her leg ulcer each day, she is to have an oral morphine mixture for pain relief. She is to have 12 mg of morphine from the available stock of 2 mg/ml. What volume of mixture should be poured for her?

2 Mrs Jones, your elderly client, is to have 8 ounces (237 ml) of Osmolite every three hours. If the drop factor for the Osmolite line is 14 drops/ml, and this feed is to last for one hour, how fast should it drip?

3 You are aware that Vitamin C is necessary for the formation of collagen, thus aiding wound healing. Mrs Jones is to have 2 g/day, to be given 6-hourly. From the available stock of 500 mg flavoured tablets, calculate the number of tablets for a single dose of medication.

4 a Mrs Jones has had a 'weak heart' for several years. She takes an oral diuretic, frusemide 40 mg each morning to help rid her body of accumulated fluids. Medication that is available and suitable for her at present is a mixture containing the equivalent of 0.01g/ml. What is the concentration of this medication in mg/ml?

   b With reference to the question above (4a), how much mixture should she be given?

5   She also has 0.25 mg of Lanoxin, a medication to slow and strengthen her heart beat. The only medication available and suitable for her is a peadiatric elixir, 50 mcg/ml. What volume of this elixir should be poured for her?

6   **a** Mrs Jones complains of a headache. She can have 0.6 g of dispersible aspirin. Stock available is 300 mg tablets, which are to be dissolved in 30 ml of water. What should she be given?

   b What is the concentration (mg per ml) of the aspirin solution in question 6a?

7   Mrs Jones's 12.00 tube feed is in progress. It is dripping at 50 drops/min and 200 ml remain in the bottle. You have been told to take your 30-minute lunch break. How long will this feed last (drop factor is 14 drops/ml) and do you have time for lunch before it completes?

8   Her leg ulcer becomes infected. Mrs Jones is commenced on the oral antibiotic Ceclor. She is to have 750 mg/day in three equally divided doses. How many mg should she have per dose?

9   Stock available is 250 mg sachets to which you are instructed to add 45 ml of tap water to make a total volume of 50 ml. How many sachets should she be given for a single dose of this medication?

10   Mrs Jones's ulcer is slow to heal. She is to take Zinc 750 mg each day for the next two weeks. Stock available is Zinvit C in 250 mg tablets. This medication is to be taken three times per day. State the number of tablets for a single dose.

11   Protein is also an essential nutrient for healing. The recommended daily intake for adults is 0.75 g/kg of ideal body/weight. Mrs Jones is 162 cm tall and weighs 44 kg. Her ideal weight is 52 kg. How much protein should she have each day?

12   **a** Each 8 ounce (237 ml) bottle of Osmolite contains 8.8 g of protein. Mrs Jones has six 3-hourly feeds, resting after her 21.00 feed until 06.00 next morning. How much protein is she having each day?

   b Does her intake of this nutrient meet the recommended daily intake?

13 You are to increase Mrs Jones's fluid intake. She is to have 60 ml of water introduced into the tube at the completion of each feed. Taking into account her tube feeds and medications, what would be her approximate daily fluid intake?

Mrs Jones's condition improves, she gains weight, feels stronger, and her ulcers begin to heal. She resumes an oral intake of her medications and nutrition.

14 Her morning frusemide is due. She is to have 40 mg and stock available is 20 mg tablets. Calculate the number of tablets she should be given.

15 Her Lanoxin is also due. She is to have 125 mcg BD. The only stock available are 62.5 mcg tablets. How many tablets should she be given per dose?

16 You are replacing Mrs Jones's morning fluid jug. She asks for orange cordial instead of water. Instructions on the cordial bottle say that the strength of cordial required is 15%. Make up 1 L of cordial at 15% strength, and state the amount of water required to complete this task.

17 You weigh Mrs Jones. Her weight is 49.5 kg. What percentage is her weight gain?

18 As the leg ulcer heals, the Vitamin C dosage is reduced to 1 g/day, to be given in four equally divided doses. Taking into account the stock available (500 mg scored tablets), calculate the number of tablets for a single dose.

EXTRA PRACTICE

19 a A client is ordered 10 mcg of drug A per kg of body weight per day, to be given tds (three times per day). What is his daily dose if he weighs 60 kg?
   b How many doses of medication should he receive each day?
   c How many mcg/dose should he be given?
   d This medication is available as 0.4 mg scored tablets. How many tablets would you expect him to be given each/dose?

20 a A client has been ordered 3 L of intravenous fluid over a 24-hour period. What volume of fluid would this order deliver each hour?

b The drop factor for the giving set is 20 drops/ml. Explain what this actually means.

c How many drops/minute would deliver the above order (20 a)?

d The registered nurse arrives at this client's bedside with 10 ml of antibiotic medication that she adds to the 30 ml of solution in the burette. She asks you to calculate the rate of flow for this new solution which is to infuse over a 10-minute period. How fast should it drip?

e You have been asked to go to lunch but you are keen to put up the second bag of intravenous fluid for his client. You note that 90 ml remain in the burette and it is dripping at 40 drops per minute. Have you time for a 30-minute lunch break?

EXERCISE EIGHT

You are working with a registered nurse in an acute surgical ward and both of you are to care for four peri-operative clients. At 07.30 you are asked to prepare an intravenous infusion for Mrs Bruce who is to be transferred to the operating theatre for a Cholecystectomy at 08.00. She is to have 1 L of 0.9% sodium chloride over a 6-hour period. The giving set emits 20 drops per ml.

1 You are to begin by 'priming the line'. What is involved in this task, and state its purpose.

2 a If the infusion is to last for 6 hours, what volume of fluid should be run into the burette each hour?

b When you examine the burette you note that the total volume of the chamber is 100 ml. Will this influence the volume you will need to put into the burette each hour, and if so, how will you manage this situation?

3 a While waiting for the infusion to be connected, you calculate the rate of flow, in drops/minute that is required. How many drops/minute will fulfil this order?

b The infusion is connected and you are regulating the flow rate. You begin by estimating the number of drops over a 15-second period. How many drops would you expect over the 15 seconds?

Mrs Collins is day two, following a Hysterectomy. On checking her notes, you observe that her 1 L 5% dextrose infusion is to complete in eight hours. You note that it was commenced at 03.00 this morning. It is now 08.30.

4 If this infusion is running to schedule, at what time would you expect it to complete?

5 a 450 ml remain in the bag and it is dripping at 36 drops/minute via a drop factor of 20 drops/ml. Is it infusing as ordered?
   b How many drops/minute should you expect to see for this order?

Ms White is also to have an infusion line prepared and commenced. She is scheduled for an Appendicectomy at 09.30. Her order is for 1 L of 0.9% sodium chloride over a 10-hour period.

6 a What volume of fluid/hour is required for this order?
   b If the drop factor for the giving set is 20 drops/ml, how fast should it drip per minute?

Miss Jones is day two following surgery to remove a tumour from her bowel. When you visit her, inspection of her intravenous infusion reveals two lines in place, her main fluid line with a smaller bag connected to the main line. The drop factor for both lines is 20 drops/ml.

8 What is this second line known as, and what is its purpose?
   a The main line is connected to a 1 L bag of 0.9% sodium chloride. What is the common name for this solution?
   b This 1 L bag of 0.9% sodium chloride is to infuse at the rate of 167 ml/hour. How long would you expect it to last?
   c When you count the drops/minute, you note that the rate of flow is 45 drops/minute. How many ml/hour will be delivered from this rate of flow?
   d How fast should Miss Jones's infusion be dripping?

9 The secondary line, containing an antibiotic, is dripping at the rate of 33 drops per minute. If both lines are delivering fluid at

the ordered rate of flow, how many ml/hour would Miss Jones currently be receiving?

10 It is 10.30 and you have been asked to take your morning tea break but you would like to change Mrs Collins's infusion on completion of the current bag. 90 ml remain in the bag and it is dripping at 56 drops/minute. Have you time for a 20-minute tea break first?

At 11.00 Ms White returns to the ward from Recovery. Her infusion is dripping at the rate of 35 drops/minute. A morphine infusion is to be set up to control her pain. The two registered nurses setting up this apparatus ask you if you would like to observe this activity.

11 But first, is the original infusion dripping at an acceptable rate of flow for her given order (Q 6b)?

12 50 mg of morphine is required for the infusion, and stock available in the ward is 10 mg/ml. What volume of morphine is required for this task?

13 This medicated infusion is to be delivered via a PCA (Patient Controlled Analgesia) machine, and the concentration of the solution is to be 1 mg of morphine to 1 ml of fluid. What would be the total volume of fluid in the syringe at the completion of this task?

14 How much solvent (normal saline) is required to complete this task?

15 Ms White is informed that she is the only person permitted to press the 'demand button' to deliver the dose of morphine. Why would this be so?

Mrs Bruce returns to the ward from Recovery at 12.30. When you have settled her into the ward, you check her intravenous infusion and note that the infusion is dripping at 58 drops per minute and 150 ml remain in the bag. A medicated infusion of pethidine, 300 mg in 100 ml of 0.9% sodium chloride, is in progress as a secondary line, via a volumetric pump.

16 Is the main infusion running to schedule?

17   The registered nurse asks you what volume of fluid should be delivered every hour if the 100 ml of the pethidine infusion is to last for 20 hours.

18   How many mg of pethidine is Mrs Bruce receiving every four hours?

19   If the recommended dose of intravenous pethidine for Mrs Bruce is 25 to 50 mg every 3 to 4 hours, is the ordered dose within these limits?

20   What is a major side effect of a narcotic infusion that you would be observing for when caring for Mrs Bruce?

You now have had time to practice nursing calculations related to intravenous fluid management and nasogastric tube feeds, so it is time to test your skills in this area. Go to the Practical Nursing Calculations website (see p. x) and complete the given calculations in Module Two, Assessments Three, Four and Five. Remember, a 100% pass is required.

EXERCISE NINE

PARENTERAL MEDICATIONS

Many medications are given by injection, either subcutaneous (SC), intramuscular (IM), or intravenous (IV). The amount (volume) of medication that will be drawn up into the syringe is dependent on what is ordered by the medical officer and what stock is available for use. Medications for injection could be available as fluid in a glass ampoule where access is gained by snapping off the top, or as powder in a glass vial (bottle) fitted with a rubber seal, held in place by a metal rim. In this case, the fluid can be accessed by a needle or fine tube called an interlink connection, inserted into the rubber cap.

A formula may be used to determine the correct dose or volume and this formula is the same as the one previously given for working out oral mixtures or medication doses.

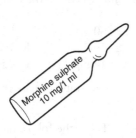

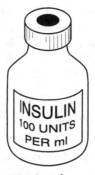

Figure 2.6 *An ampoule*   **Figure 2.7** *A vial*

Formula

$$\frac{\text{Strength required}}{\text{Strength available}} \times \frac{\text{Volume in which available strength is dissolved}}{1}$$

Example

Mr Timson is to have 60 mg of pethidine for pain relief. Stock available is 100 mg/2 ml.

$$\frac{60 \text{ mg}}{50 \text{ mg}} \times \frac{1 \text{ ml (Vol)}}{1} = \frac{60}{50} = \frac{6}{5} \text{ or } 1.2 \text{ ml}$$

Activity

Complete the following by indicating on the syringe below, the volume to be drawn up.

1 a Medication required is
      40 mg
      Stock available is 30 mg/ml

   b Medication required is
      60 mg
      Stock available is 30 mg/ml

   c Medication required is
      75 mg
      Stock available is 100 mg/2 ml

2   From available stock of 100 mg/2 ml, calculate the following
    required doses of medication.
    a 40 mg   b 20 mg   c 60 mg   d 50 mg
    e 10 mg   f 80 mg   g 30 mg   h 70 mg
    i 15 mg   j 90 mg   k 75 mg   l 25 mg

Note: some medication is measured in units rather than mg, for
example insulin.

3   Medication required is 200 000 units. From the following avail-
    able stocks, calculate the volume of this dose.
    a 100 000 units/ml   b 200 000 units/ml
    c 500 000 units/ml   d 50 000 units/ml
    e 250 000 units/ml   f 400 000 units/ml

4   You have stock on hand of 10 mcg/2 ml. Calculate the following
    required volumes of medication from this stock.
    a 2 mcg   b 8 mcg   c 14 mcg   d 10 mcg
    e 3 mcg   f 12 mcg   g 7 mcg   h 9 mcg
    i 2.5 mcg   j 5 mcg   k 4 mcg   l 6 mcg

5   You have stock on hand of 10 mg/ml. Calculate the required
    volumes for the following medication orders.
    a 0.006 g   b 7 mg   c 5 mg   d 0.025 g
    e 2 mg   f 12 mg   g 10 mg   h 8 mg
    i 1 mg   j 3 mg   k 4 mg   l 9 mg

6   You have stock on hand of 5000 units/0.2 ml. Calculate the
    required volumes for the following medication orders. Indicate
    the type of syringe that would be most appropriate for these
    orders.
    a 2500 units   b 5000 units   c 7500 units   d 10 000 units
    e 3000 units   f 4000 units   g 6000 units   h 8000 units

MIXING MEDICATED SOLUTIONS

Some medications that are in use are available only in powder form.
These medications need to be mixed with sterile water or normal
saline to form a solution that can be drawn up and injected.

These medications are unstable if left in solution for too long a
period, hence, they are mixed with a solvent just prior to use.

Manufacturing instructions accompanying the medication and pharmacological texts such as MIMS will tell you how much solvent to add in order to obtain the concentration required. These instructions will also indicate the type of fluid that should be used. The powder in the vial *must always* be taken into account when reconstituting (or making up) the medication *if the dose to be given is less than the total volume*. For example, 250 mg may be ordered for a child from a vial containing one gram. When the powder is mixed with fluid it will increase the volume of the given fluid because the powder occupies space, thus it is essential that the powder is considered, to ensure an accurate dose.

 ## Example

1 gram of powder (drug X) in a 10 ml vial has to be reconstituted or made into a solution with a concentration of 100 mg/ml. This means that every ml of fluid in solution will contain 100 mg of drug X. The total volume of this medication will be the total dose (1000 mg), divided by the dose (100 mg) per ml. So 1000 mg ÷ 100 mg/ml is 10 ml of fluid.

Suppose that this 1 gram of powder displaces 1 ml of fluid when a solution is formed. This would mean that the fluid volume of 10 ml would be made up of 9 ml of solvent (the sterile water or saline that you have just added) plus the 1 gram of powder or solute. Thus, when making up this solution of 100 mg/ml, 9 ml of fluid would be added to the vial.

To reiterate this point. Together, the one gram of powder (solute) and the 9 ml of sterile water (solvent) make up the solution (of 10 ml) containing 100 mg of drug X per ml. This is a w/v ratio.

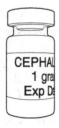

CEPHA
1 gra
Exp D

Figure 2.8 *10 ml vial showing 1 gram of antibiotic powder which occupies the space of 1 ml of fluid*

The vial in Fig. 2.8 has the capacity to hold 10 ml of fluid when in solution. Consider the contents of the vial and note the space that the powder occupies and then calculate the amount of fluid that would be required to reconstitute this medication to a concentration of 100 mg per 1 ml of fluid as the example above.

Table 2.1 *An example of dilution guidelines for the medication ampicillin sodium*

Label strength	Recommended amount sterile water for injections BP	Final concentration
500 mg	1.7 ml	250 mg/ml
	2.2 ml	200 mg/ml
	4.7 ml	100 mg/ml
1 g	1.3 ml	500 mg/ml
	3.3 ml	250 mg/ml
	9.3 ml	100 mg/ml

Source: MIMS, 2001, 8–612; reproduced with permission of MIMS Australia

Activity

7 Assume that the powdered form of drug H is 1 000 000 units and it displaces 1.4 ml of fluid. Reconstitute to the following concentrations by indicating the volume of fluid necessary to make the required solution of drug H.

   a 100 000 units/ml   **b** 200 000 units/ml
   c 500 000 units/ml   **d** 50 000 units/ml
   e 250 000 units/ml   **f** 400 000 units/ml

8 1 gram of powdered drug J displaces 1 ml of fluid. Indicate the volume of fluid required to reconstitute drug J to the following concentrations.

   a 200 mg/ml   **b** 250 mg/ml
   c 500 mg/ml   **d** 50 mg/ml
   e 100 mg/ml   **f** 400 mg/ml

9 1 gram of ampicillin sodium will displace 0.7 ml of fluid when reconstitution occurs. Indicate the volume of fluid required to reconstitute this medication to the following concentrations.

> **a** 50 mg/ml   **b** 100 mg/ml
> **c** 200 mg/ml   **d** 250 mg/ml
> **e** 25 mg/ml   **f** 500 mg/ml

10 A client has been ordered 2 grams of ampicillin sodium per day, to be given in four equally divided doses. Calculate a single dose of medication for this person.

11 Ampicillin sodium is available as 1 gram of powder in a 10 ml vial, and accompanying instructions indicate that the powder will occupy 0.7 ml of the reconstituted solution. What volume of sterile water is required to obtain a concentration of 250 mg/ml?

12 Following reconstitution with a concentration of 250 mg/ml, what volume of solution will need to be drawn up for his first dose?

13 **a** A client has been ordered 10 mcg of drug A, per kg of body weight per day, to be given QID. If she weighs 60 kg, what is her daily dose of this medication?

     b With reference to Q 13a, how many mcg should she be given for a single dose?

     c Stock available is 200 mcg/ml, what volume should be drawn up for the above medication?

14 A client is ordered 300 units of drug B per hour, for 24 hours, to be added to 500 ml of an 0.9% sodium chloride infusion. How many units of drug B will be necessary to fulfil this order?

15 Stock available for the above order (Q 14) is 25 000 units/ml. What volume will need to be drawn up, and what type of syringe would be most accurate for this task?

16 A volumetric pump is to be used to fulfil this order. How fast will the above solution need to infuse to deliver the required dose in the given time?

17 A client is ordered 1 gram of drug C. Instructions accompanying the medication advise you to add 9.3 ml of sterile water to achieve a concentration of 100 mg/ml. What volume of fluid has the 1 gram of medication displaced?

18 This medication is to be added to 40 ml of intravenous fluid already in the burette, and infused over a 20-minute period. If the drop factor for the giving set is 20 drops/ml, how fast should this medicated solution drip?

19 a A client is ordered 25 mg/kg of body weight of drug D per day, to be given 4/24. If his weight is 60 kg, what is his daily dose of this medication?

b How many doses per day does the figure '4/24' denote?

c How many mg is in a single dose of this medication?

d Stock available is 0.25 g capsules. What should he be given for a single dose?

20 a A client has a medicated infusion with 400 mg of drug E dissolved in 100 ml. This medicated infusion is to last for 20 hours. How many ml/hour should be delivered?

b How many mg of drug E is this client receiving every 4 hours?

 # EXERCISE TEN

You are caring for Ms Sally Boyer, a 25-year-old woman, who has been transferred from a small country hospital with a severe chest infection. Sally's notes indicate that she has a past history of Bronchitis and Pleurisy and she regularly smokes approximately 25 cigarettes each day.

On admission she is febrile, dyspnoeic, flushed, lethargic and has a productive cough with green-coloured sputum. She tells you that her chest feels tight. A diagnosis of right Lobar Pneumonia is made. Oxygen, at 8 L/minute is commenced and an intravenous line is established. The first 1 L of sodium chloride is to infuse over a 6-hour period.

1 How many ml/hour should Sally receive from this infusion?

2 If the drop factor for the giving set is 20 drops/ml, to what rate of flow (in drops/min) should the infusion be regulated?

An antibiotic regime is commenced immediately to help combat Sally's chest infection. At 08.00 intravenous ceftriaxone sodium (Rocephin) 2 grams is ordered, to be given daily. Stock available is a 10 ml vial containing 1 gram of powder. Instructions accompanying the medication indicate that you should mix the powder with 9 ml of sterile water for reconstitution.

3 What volume of fluid should the registered nurse draw up for this morning dose?

4 This medicated solution is to be added to the 30 ml of fluid in the burette and infused over a 15-minute period. To what rate of flow (in drops/minute) should you adjust the giving set?

4 grams/day of intravenous erythromycin is to be given 6-hourly and is to commence at 10.00. It is available as 1 gram of powder in a 10 ml vial. Accompanying instructions indicate that the 1 g of powder will displace 1 ml of fluid when reconstituted.

5 How many mg of erythromycin should Sally receive for a single dose?

6 If the reconstituted medication has a concentration of 100 mg/ml, what volume should be drawn up for a single dose?

7 The concentration of this medication when infused is to be no greater than 10 mg/ml of fluid. How much fluid will need to be added to the burette to achieve this concentration?

8 When the required amount of fluid is added to the burette and combined with the medication, to what rate of flow (in drops per minute) will you adjust the giving set to complete this administration in 40 minutes?

Sally reminds you that her chest is very tight and that it hurts her to breathe. She asks you for some pain relief medication. She is seen by the medical officer who orders subcutaneous morphine.

9 Sally is permitted 7.5 mg of morphine. Stock available is 15 mg/ml, so what volume should you draw up?

10 You are to give Sally 5 mg of salbutamol (Ventolin). This medication is available as a solution, 5 mg/ml. She is to have this inhalation at a 1:1 (V/V) ratio with sterile sodium chloride. How much sodium chloride is required for this task?

Sally's condition remains poor. She is refusing fluids and food, continues to be febrile and her breathing difficulties persist. The oral antibiotic roxithromycin (Biaxsig), 300 mg/day, is to be given BD. As this medication needs to be taken prior to meals, it is routinely given at 07.30 and 17.00. Because Sally has not eaten recently, it is commenced at 13.00.

11 Stock in the ward is 150 mg tablets. How many tablets should you give her?

12 While doing your routine observations for 14.00, you note that her oxygen saturation level has dropped to 87%. You report these findings and the flow of oxygen is increased to 12 L/minute. What percentage increase is the oxygen now, compared to her admission order?

13 Sally calls you and tells you that she is 'going to be sick'. You check her notes and see that metoclopramide (Maxolon) 10 mg may be given PRN for nausea or vomiting. Do any of her current medications note nausea and vomiting as a side effect?

14 Stock of Maxolon on hand is an ampoule containing 10 mg/2 ml. What volume should be drawn up?

15 At 13.00 you are asked to go to lunch. Because you are keen to put up the second bag of intravenous fluid, you decide to check what time you need to be back in the ward. If 150 ml remain in the bag and it is dripping at 60 drops per minute, have you time for a 30-minute lunch break?

16 How many ml/hour is being infused if the rate of flow is 60 drops/minute?

17 In relation to Q 1, how much fluid/hour should Sally be receiving?

18 At 14.00 her second bag of fluid, 5% dextrose is commenced and is to last for 8 hours. How many ml/hour will she receive from this order?

19 How many drops/minute will deliver this order?

20 When checking her medication chart you notice that temazepam (Normison) 10 mg has been ordered nocte to help her to relax and sleep. If stock in the ward is equivalent to 0.01 g/tablet, how many tablets would you expect her to be given?

You have now completed your first year of a nursing degree. There is an expectation that you will be competent in *all* the nursing calculations that you have been taught to date. It is time to return to the Practical Nursing Calculations website (see p. x) to assess your knowledge by completing the questions in Module Two, Assessments Six and Seven in the allotted time of 20 minutes each. Once again a 100% pass is expected. If you still find that you are unable to achieve the 100% pass, perhaps it is time to review these areas by going back to earlier chapters and re-doing areas that continue to cause concern. Extra work is available on the website for use as required.

 # ANSWERS

EXERCISE ONE

1 **a** 1/2 tablet   **b** $1\frac{1}{2}$ tablets   **c** 2 tablets   **d** $2\frac{1}{2}$ tablets

2 **a** 2 tablets   **b** 1/2 tablet   **c** 4 tablets   **d** 1 tablet

3 **a** 1 tablet   **b** 1/2 tablet   **c** 2 tablets   **d** 3 tablets

4 **a** $1\frac{1}{2} \times 50$ mg **b** 1×50 mg, 1×20 mg, 1×10 mg, or 4×20 mg

    c $1\frac{1}{2} \times 10$ mg **d** 1×100 mg, 1×50 mg

5 **a** 1/4 tablet   **b** 1 tablet   **c** 1/2 tablet   **d** 1 tablet

6 **a** 2 tablets   **b** 1 tablet   **c** 1 tablet   **d** 1/2 tablet

7 **a** 1 tablet   **b** 1 tablet   **c** $1\frac{1}{2}$ tablets **d** 2 tablets

8 **a** 1/2 tablet   **b** 1/2 tablet   **c** 1/2 tablet   **d** $1\frac{1}{2}$ tablets

9 **a** 1/4 tablet   **b** 1/2 tablet   **c** 2 tablets   **d** 3 tablets

10 **a** 1 tablet   **b** 2 tablets   **c** 1 tablet   **d** 2 tablets

11 1/2 tablet

12 2 tablets

13 1/4 tablet

14 1/2 tablet

15 **a** 500 mg/dose   **b** 2 capsules

16 **a** 25 mcg/dose   **b** 1/2 tablet/dose

17 **a** 500 mg/dose   **b** 2 capsules/dose

18 **a** 40 mg/dose   **b** 2 tablets/dose

19 **a** 500 mg/dose   **b** 1 capsule/dose

20 **a** 100 mg/dose   **b** 1 tablet/dose

EXERCISE TWO

$$\frac{\text{Dose prescribed}}{\text{Stock strength}} \times \frac{\text{Volume in which available strength is dissolved}}{1}$$

1	**a** 6 ml	**b** 4 ml	**c** 5 ml	**d** 5 ml
	e 5 ml	**f** 8 ml	**g** 8 ml	**h** 3 ml
2	**a** 20 ml	**b** 2 ml	**c** 25 ml	**d** 8 ml
	e 4 ml	**f** 7.5 ml	**g** 5 ml	**h** 25 ml
3	**a** 12 ml	**b** 8 ml	**c** 8 ml	**d** 3 ml
	e 15 ml	**f** 6 ml	**g** 9 ml	**h** 1 ml
4	**a** 2.5 ml	**b** 1.2 ml	**c** 3 ml	**d** 5 ml
	e 12 ml	**f** 2 ml	**g** 5 ml	**h** 1 ml

$$\frac{\text{Volume prescribed}}{\text{Volume available}} \times \frac{\text{Dose contained in volume available}}{1}$$

5 **a** 250 mg   **b** Dose is fine, $10 \times 25 = 250$

6 **a** 400 mg   **b** Yes, it is within limits, $\frac{8}{10}$ of $500 = 400$

7 **a** 240 mg   **b** Yes, $20 \times 12.5 = 250$

8 **a** 60 mg   **b** Yes, $\frac{6}{10} \times 100 = 60$

9 800 mg/day

10 200 mg/dose

11 8 ml

12 240 mg

13 Yes, $15 \times 20 = 300$

14 1600 ml

15 160 ml

16 12.5 ml

17 96 mg/day

18 48 mg/dose

19 6 ml

20 **a** 150 ml/hour   **b** 100 ml/hour

EXERCISE THREE

1 **a** 192 mg   **b** 6 ml   **c** $1\frac{1}{2}$ tablets   **d** 2 tablets

   e 8 ml   **f** 15 ml   **g** 20 ml   **h** 2 tablets

   i $1\frac{1}{2}$ tablets   **j** 3 tablets

2 **a** 160 cm   **b** 44.55 kg

3 **a** 500 mg/dose **b** 1 tablet/dose

4 0.5 mg/day

5 **a** 5 days   **b** 200 mcg/bottle

6 **a** 1422 ml   **b** 360 ml

7 3318 drops/237 ml

8 55 drops/minute

9   3.95 ml/minute

10   Yes

11   **a**   2 ml/minute   **b**   Almost 2 hours (118.5 min)

12   5 ml

13   20 ml

14   **a**   180 ml   **b**   1 to 9 or 1 in 10   **c**   0.1

15   2 tablets

16   20 ml of 0.9% solution

17   40 ml

18   1/2 tablet/dose

19   250 mg

20   $1\frac{1}{2}$ tablets

EXERCISE FOUR

1   $1.673

2   $5.79

3   $3.12

4   $6.20

5   $0.41

6   $2.97

7   $20.16

8   $100.80

9   $2688

10   $981 120

11   65% survive

12   Approximately 8896

13   2732

14 37 680

15 9277

16 **a** 0.75 grams   **b** 2.25 grams   **c** $1\frac{1}{2}$ tablets

17 **a** 3600   **b** $\dfrac{30 \text{ drops/minute}}{20 \text{ drops/ml}} \times \dfrac{60 \text{ minutes}}{1} = 90$ ml/hour

   c 2 hours

18 **a** 5 mg/ml   **b** 6.25 days

19 **a** 10 ml   **b** 6 ml

20 **a** 250 mcg   **b** 2 tablets

EXERCISE FIVE

1 **a** 150 ml/hour, 50 dpm   **b** 100 ml/hour, 25 dpm
   c 200 ml/hour, 67 dpm

2 **a** 80 ml/hr   **b** 75 ml/hr   **c** 100 ml/hr
   d 250 ml/hr   **e** 150 ml/hr   **f** 50 ml/hr

3 **a** 62–63 dpm   **b** 50 dpm   **c** 85 dpm
   d 80 dpm   **e** 50 dpm   **f** 100 dpm

4 **a** 50 dpm   **b** 50 dpm   **c** 55–56 dpm
   d 33 dpm   **e** 50 dpm   **f** 50 dpm

5 **a** 25 dpm   **b** 37–38 dpm   **c** 44 dpm
   d 19 dpm   **e** 28 dpm   **f** 20 dpm

6 **a** 17 dpm   **b** 20 dpm   **c** 23 dpm
   d 25 dpm   **e** 33 dpm   **f** 100 dpm

7 **a** 50 dpm   **b** 50 dpm   **c** 60 dpm
   d 80 dpm   **e** 27 dpm   **f** 100 dpm

8 **a** 45 dpm   **b** 50 dpm   **c** 30 dpm
   d 60 dpm   **e** 25 dpm   **f** 45 dpm

9 **a** 60 dpm   **b** 45 dpm   **c** 45 dpm
   d 60 dpm   **e** 40 dpm   **f** 30 dpm

10   a   30 dpm   b   30 dpm   c   40 dpm
      d   40 dpm   e   45 dpm   f   47 dpm

11   a   50 minutes   b   80 minutes   c   86 minutes
      d   52 minutes

12   a   60 minutes   b   60 minutes   c   30 minutes
      d   45 minutes

13   a   175 ml/hour   b   110 ml/hour   c   133 ml/hour
      d   192 ml/hour

14   a   3 ml/minute   b   2 ml/minute   c   0.5 ml/minute
      d   1 ml/minute   e   0.75 ml/minute
      f   2.5 ml/minute

15   a   0.5 ml/minute   b   0.33 ml/minute
      c   0.25 ml/minute   d   0.75 ml/minute
      e   1 ml/minute   f   1.25 ml/minute

16   a   120 ml/hour   b   120 ml/hour   c   45 ml/hour
      d   150 ml/hour   e   240 ml/hour   f   30 ml/hour

17   a   125 ml/hour and 42 drops/minute
      b   20 drops/minute

18   a   145 ml/hour   b   150 ml/hour for the third hour
      c   120 minutes

19   a   35 drops/min   b   23 drops/min   c   54 drops/min
      d   21 drops/min   e   12 drops/ml   f   39 drops/min

20   a   29 drops/min   b   17–18 drops/min
      c   12 drops/min   d   70 drops/min
      e   87–88 drops/min   f   93 drops/min

EXERCISE SIX

1   a   240 mg   b   6.7 ml   c   1/2 tablet   d   1 tablet
      e   10 ml   f   10 ml   g   9 ml   h   2 tablets
      i $1\frac{1}{2}$ tablets   j   2 tablets

2 1/2 tablet

3 2 tablets

4 2 ml

5 98 ml

6 Yes, she may have the 2 tablets

7 0.9 g

8 80 kg

9 Approx 188 cm

10 8000 kilojoules

11 2056 ml

12 3318 potential drops

13 55 drops/minute

14 250 mg/dose

15 1 capsule/dose

16 $1\frac{1}{2}$ tablets

17 660 mg

18 1 tablet

19 40 ml of iced water

20 20% is water

EXERCISE SEVEN

1 6 ml

2 55 drops/minute

3 1 tablet

4 **a** 10 mg/ml   **b** 4 ml/dose

5   5 ml/dose

6   **a** 2 tablets   **b** 20 mg/ml

7   Yes, the feed should complete in 56 minutes

8   250 mg/dose

9   Use one sachet plus 45 ml of water

10   1 tablet/dose

11   39 grams/day

12   **a** 52.8 grams   **b** Yes, 39 grams was the recommended amount

13   Approximately 1962 ml including medications

14   2 tablets

15   2 tablets

16   850 ml of water

17   12.5%

18   1/2 tablet

19   **a** 600 mcg   **b** 3 doses per day
     c 200 mcg/dose   **d** 1/2 tablet/dose

20   **a** 125 ml/hour
     b Every ml that leaves the giving set comprises 20 drops
     c 42 drops/minute
     d 80 drops/minute
     e Yes, 90 ml × 20 drops/ml ÷ 40 drops/minute = 45 minutes

EXERCISE EIGHT

1   Priming the line is a procedure to remove all the air from the line
    before it is connected via a vein into the circulatory system. If air
    enters the circulatory system, it could cause a life-threatening air
    embolus.

2   **a** 167 ml/hour
    b Fill the burette to 83 ml every 30 minutes or fill it to 100 ml
    and return in 30 minutes to add 67 ml. Any action is accept-

able so long as the correct volume is added and the fluid does not run out in the burette.

3 **a** 56 drops/minute **b** 14 drops every 15 seconds

4 11.00

5 **a** No, it is behind schedule, 312 ml should be in the bag
 b It should be dripping at 42 drops/min

6 **a** 100 ml/hour

 b $\dfrac{1000 \text{ (vol)}}{600 \text{ (10 hr} \times 60 \text{ min)}}$ = 1.66 ml/min × 20 d/ml = 33 dpm

7 The second line is known as a secondary or a 'piggy-back' line. It is used to deliver another solution, often a medicated solution over a shorter period of time.

8 **a** Normal saline **b** Approximately 6 hours

 c $\dfrac{45 \text{ dpm}}{20 \text{ d/ml}}$ = 2.25 ml/min × 60 = 135 ml/hr

 d 55–56 drops/minute

9 267 ml/hour 33 drops ÷ 20 drops/ml = 1.65 ml/minute × 60 = 99 ml
  56 drops ÷ 20 drops/ml = 2.8 ml/minute × 60 = 168 ml

10 Yes, this infusion should last 32 minutes

11 Slightly fast, it should be 33 drops/minute

12 5 ml of morphine analgesia

13 50 ml

14 45 ml

15 So that she alone has total control over her pain management

16 No, slightly faster than ordered

17 5 ml/hour

18 60 mg/4 hours

19 Yes, maximum dose would be 50 mg × 8 doses or 400 mg

20 Depressed or reduced breathing

EXERCISE NINE

1 **a** 1.3 ml

1.3

 b 2 ml

2

 c 1.5 ml

1.5

2	**a** 0.8 ml	**b** 0.4 ml	**c** 1.2 ml	**d** 1 ml
	e 0.2 ml	**f** 1.6 ml	**g** 0.6 ml	**h** 1.4 ml
	i 0.3 ml	**j** 1.8 ml	**k** 1.5	**l** 0.5 ml
3	**a** 2 ml	**b** 1 ml	**c** 0.4 ml	**d** 4 ml
	e 0.8 ml	**f** 0.5 ml		
4	**a** 0.4 ml	**b** 1.6 ml	**c** 2.8 ml	**d** 2 ml
	e 0.6 ml	**f** 2.4 ml	**g** 1.4 ml	**h** 1.8 ml
	i 0.5 ml	**j** 1 ml	**k** 0.8 ml	**l** 1.2 ml
5	**a** 0.6 ml	**b** 0.7 ml	**c** 0.5 ml	**d** 2.5 ml
	e 0.2 ml	**f** 1.2 ml	**g** 1 ml	**h** 0.8 ml
	i 0.1 ml	**j** 0.3 ml	**k** 0.4 ml	**l** 0.9 ml
6	**a** 0.1 ml	**b** 0.2 ml	**c** 0.3 ml	**d** 0.4 ml
	e 0.12 ml	**f** 0.16 ml	**g** 0.24 ml	**h** 0.32 ml

All require insulin syringes to be used.

7	**a** 8.6 ml	**b** 3.6 ml	**c** 0.6 ml	**d** 18.6 ml
	e 2.6 ml	**f** 1.1 ml		
8	**a** 4 ml	**b** 3 ml	**c** 1 ml	**d** 19 ml
	e 9 ml	**f** 1.5 ml		
9	**a** 19.3 ml	**b** 9.3 ml	**c** 4.3 ml	**d** 3.3 ml
	e 39.3 ml	**f** 1.3 ml		

10 500 mg

11 3.3 ml

12 2 ml

13 **a** 600 mcg   **b** 150 mcg   **c** 0.75 ml

14 7200 units

15 0.29 ml, use a 0.5 ml insulin syringe

16 20.83 ml/hour

17 0.7 ml has been displaced

18 50 drops/minute

19 a 1500 mg   b 6 doses per day
   c 250 mg/dose   d 1 capsule/dose

20 a 5 ml/hour   b 80 mg/4 hours

EXERCISE TEN

1 167 ml/hour

2 56 drops/minute

3 20 ml for the 2 grams

4 67 drops/minute

5 1000 mg/dose

6 10 ml

7 90 ml

8 50 drops/minute

9 0.5 ml

10 1 ml

11 1 tablet

12 50% increase

13 Yes, morphine can cause nausea

14 2 ml

15 Yes, the infusion should last 50 minutes

16 180 ml/hour

17   167 ml/hour

18   125 ml/hour

19   42 drops/minute

20   1 tablet

3

Advanced Medication and Intravenous Calculations

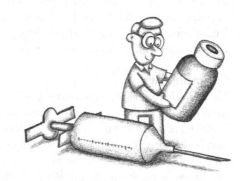

Objectives

After completing the given calculations, it is expected that you should be able to:

1 enhance the speed at which you compute previously learned calculations

2 calculate the dosages of parenteral medications, including those which require reconstitution

3 verify that dosages can be safely given

4 demonstrate the theoretical management of an intravenous infusion

5 demonstrate the theoretical management of volumetric pumps and the administration of bolus doses related to infusion pumps

EXERCISE ONE

INTRAVENOUS BOLUS DOSAGES

Intravenous medications may be given by an intravenous 'push' or a 'bolus' dose. This technique is used to administer medications that need to be given rapidly to have the desired therapeutic effect. This technique could be used to administer a slow, single dose of intravenous morphine, for example, for a person who is experiencing severe chest pain. On the other hand, a bolus dose of morphine can also be given to a person on a continuous morphine infusion where relief is required for breakthrough pain.

 ### Example One

Mrs Black, who has severe chest pain, is to have 10 mg of intravenous morphine over a 4-minute period. Stock available is 10 mg/ml. Once the 1 ml of medication is drawn up, give 2 mg (or 0.2 ml) at once and repeat every minute until the 10 mg has been pushed through as a bolus dose.

 ### Example Two

Mr Evans is receiving a continuous pethidine infusion via a volumetric infusion pump. This medicated solution contains 500 mg of pethidine in 100 ml of 0.9% sodium chloride and is to last for 25 hours. The infusion or volumetric pump is currently delivering the medication at the rate of 4 ml/hour, or 20 mg/hour. From this medicated solution, Mr Evans is receiving 20 mg of pethidine every hour. However, he states that his pain has become unbearable. An order for a bolus dose of 12 mg of pethidine over a 4-minute period has been given.

So, to what speed, in ml/hour, will you need to adjust the infusion pump to deliver the prescribed dose in the specified time? First, find the dose/minute that is required from this order:

12 mg ÷ 4 minutes = 3 mg/minute

 ### Formula

$$\frac{\text{Dose required}}{\text{Dose available}} \times \frac{\text{Volume} \times 60 \text{ minutes}}{1} \text{ or}$$

$$\frac{3 \text{ mg}}{500 \text{ mg}} \times \frac{100 \text{ ml} \times 60 \text{ minutes}}{1} = 36 \text{ ml/hour}$$

You should adjust the rate of flow to 36 ml/hour for the four minutes, and then return the rate of flow to the ordered rate of 4 ml/hour.

Activity

Calculate the volume/hour for the following bolus doses

1 500 mg of drug A in a 100 ml solution
    a 10 mg in 2 minutes   **b** 15 mg in 3 minutes
    c 18 mg in 3 minutes   **d** 12 mg in 4 minutes

2 90 mg of drug B in a 30 ml solution
    a 6 mg in 3 minutes   **b** 4.5 mg in 3 minutes
    c 8 mg in 4 minutes   **d** 4 mg in 4 minutes

3 600 mg of drug C in a 100 ml solution
    a 20 mg in 4 minutes   **b** 18 mg in 3 minutes
    c 12 mg in 4 minutes   **d** 10 mg in 4 minutes

4 60 mg of drug D in a 60 ml solution
    a 8 mg in 4 minutes   **b** 6 mg in 4 minutes
    c 4 mg in 4 minutes   **d** 6 mg in 3 minutes

5 300 mg in 100 ml of solution
    a 9 mg in 3 minutes   **b** 6 mg in 4 minutes
    c 12 mg in 3 minutes   **d** 15 mg in 3 minutes

You are caring for Mr Green, an elderly gentleman, who has a heart condition, Diabetes and a leg ulcer. While checking his medication folder prior to the morning handover, you note when his oral medications are due.

6 At 07.00 you give him his early morning diuretic, frusemide (Lasix) 40 mg. Stock available is 20 mg tablets. Calculate the number of tablets he should be given.

7 When his breakfast arrives at 08.00, his Slow K pill is due. He is to have 600 mg. From available stock equivalent to 0.6 g, how many pills should he be given?

8 What is the chemical name for Slow K?

9 Why does he need to take Slow K?

10 He asks you to crush this medication (the Slow K) as it is too difficult for him to swallow. How should you manage this situation?

11 His tolbutamide (Rastinon), a medication to assist in lowering his blood glucose level, is due as soon as his breakfast is completed. His order is for 500 mg of this medication and stock available is 1 g scored tablets. Calculate the number of tablets he should be given.

12 As you offer him his medication, his water jug is returned to him. He asks you to make up 1 L of cordial, 1 in 5 strength, from the low kilojoule cordial in his locker. How much cordial will you pour into the jug before you add the iced water?

When you offer to assist him to the shower, he asks to remain in bed for a while as he has chest pain. He asks you to pass him his glyceryl trinitrate (Anginine) tablets. You note that these tablets help to relieve angina pain by causing vasodilation, and instructions on the bottle say that he can have a maximum of three tablets or 1.8 mg in a 10-minute period for severe pain.

13 What is the dose, in mcg, of each tablet?

14 At 10.00 his lanoxin (Digoxin), a medication to slow and strengthen cardiac contractions, is due. His order is for 0.25 mg. The only stock currently available on the ward is 125 mcg tablets. How many tablets should he be given?

15 Nifedipine (Adalat), a potent coronary and peripheral vasodilator, is also due at 10.00. It is available in 20 mg tablets or 10 mg capsules. What should you give this gentleman to fulfil his order for 20 mg?

It is 09.30 and you are to clean and redress the ulcer on Mr Green's leg. As part of your assessment for this procedure you ask him if he requires pain relief prior to the dressing. He tells you it is a very painful procedure and he wants his 'usual tablets'.

16 His medication order states that he can have oral methadone (Physeptone) 20 mg, PRN prior to his dressing change. Stock available is 10 mg tablets. Calculate the number of tablets you should give him.

17 While pouring him a glass of cordial for this medication you notice that he has a packet of Disprin capsules in his locker

drawer. Does this medication have any significance in relation to any of his current medications?

18 The leg ulcer is cleaned with 0.9% sodium chloride. How many mg of salt is in this 50 ml solution? Assessment of the ulcer indicates that an infection is present. The medical officer prescribes ampicillin 2 g per day, to be given 6-hourly.

19 Calculate a single dose of this medication.

20 How many 250 mg capsules should he be given for his first dose of this medication?

 EXERCISE TWO

You are on the late shift and have been asked to care for sixteen-year-old Monique who has been admitted to the ward for an elective Appendicectomy in the morning.

1 At 21.00 she asks for something to help her to sleep. Nitrazepam (Mogadon) 10 mg is ordered. If stock available is equivalent to 0.005 g, how many tablets should she be given?

When you return to duty next morning, you are again assigned to care for Monique. After fasting from 24.00, she is to have her premedication at 07.30. She is to have pethidine 60 mg and atropine sulphate 0.3 mg.

2 Calculate the volume of pethidine she should receive if stock available is 100 mg/2 ml.

3 Atropine sulphate is available as 600 mcg/ml. What volume should you draw up?

4 a Monique returns to the ward at 11.00. An intravenous line with 1 L of 0.9% sodium chloride is in progress, dripping at 40 drops/minute. If the drop factor for the giving set is 20 drops/ml, how many ml per minute is she receiving?
   b How many ml/hour is the set delivering?

5 If the 1 L bag of intravenous fluid commenced at 08.00, and continues at its current rate of flow, at what time would you expect it to complete?

At 12.00 a continuous pethidine infusion is to commence. It is to contain 300 mg of pethidine in a 100 ml bag of 0.9% sodium chloride. The two registered nurses carrying out this task ask you to complete the required calculations to enhance your mathematical skills.

6 a If stock available is pethidine 100 mg/2 ml, what volume of pethidine is required for this task?

  b To maintain a total volume of 100 ml of 0.9% of sodium chloride, how much fluid will need to be removed from the bag to accommodate the pethidine?

7 What is the concentration (in mg/ml) of this medicated solution?

8 The pethidine solution is connected to Monique's infusion via a volumetric pump, using a secondary line, and is to last for 25 hours. How much pethidine per hour will Monique receive?

9 At what rate (in ml/hr) should the volumetric pump be set?

At 13.00 Monique asks for 'something stronger' as her pain is quite intense. She is ordered a bolus dose of 12 mg of pethidine over a 4-minute period.

10 How many mg/minute should she receive from this bolus dose?

11 Bearing in mind the concentration of this medicated solution, how many ml of fluid will deliver to her this dose per minute?

12 Remembering that the fluid that you have just calculated is for one minute only, to what rate of flow, in ml/hour, will you need to adjust the volumetric pump to deliver 12 mg in four minutes?

13 Taking into account the bolus dose that Monique has just received, what is the revised time for this pethidine infusion to complete?

At 16.20 her second intravenous bag of fluid, 1 L of 4% dextrose in 0.18% sodium chloride is commenced and is to last for ten hours.

14 a Calculate the volume per hour that she should receive from the bag.

  b How many drops/minute should deliver the above volume?

Next morning when you arrive in the ward, you are asked to care for Monique again. You visit her after handover at 07.30 and note that her third intravenous bag of fluid, 1 L of 0.9% sodium chloride which commenced at 02.30 this morning, is to infuse over a 12-hour period.

15 At what speed (in drops/minute) should this infusion be dripping?

16 590 ml remain in the bag. Is it running to schedule?

Following assessment which indicates that bowel sounds are present, Monique is permitted oral fluids. At 10.00 she may have 40 ml/hour which is to continue until 20.00.

17 If she drinks all of this fluid, how much oral fluid will be charted on her intake chart?

18 At 12.00 the pethidine infusion pump is removed on completion. In relation to this infusion, how much fluid will be charted on the intake column for day two?

19 As Monique is tolerating oral fluids, her intravenous line is discontinued on completion of the current bag at 14.30. Using the fluid balance chart supplied (see Fig. 3.1), fill in and total her intake for day two (midnight to midnight).

20 It is day three and Monique is ready for discharge. She may have one Panadeine tablet every four hours for pain for the next 48 hours. How many tablets should the pharmacy dispense?

EXERCISE THREE

It is 16.30 and Mrs Ferris has just been admitted to the ward for a Cholecystectomy in the morning. As she is settled for the night, she requests sedation.

1 She is ordered nitrazepam (Mogadon) 10 mg to help her to sleep. If stock available is equivalent to 0.01 g, calculate the number of tablets she should be given.

It is 07.00 on the day of Mrs Ferris's operation and as you are caring for her today, you are to prepare her premedication of 16 mg of papaveretum (Omnopon) and 400 mcg of hyoscine.

						FLUID BALANCE CHART				

Ward

FLINDERS MEDICAL CENTRE

FLUID BALANCE CHART

Surname SMART

Other Names Monique Helen

D.O.B./Sex 6 – 7 - 1987 female

Medical Officer:	Date:

Address

Medi. No. 567 891 234

	INTAKE				OUTPUT					
Time	By Mouth or Tube (Description)	ml	Intravenous	ml	Vomitus or Aspirate	ml	Faeces and Other Drainage (Description)	ml	Urine ml
0100									
0200									
0300									
0400									
0500									
0600									
0700									
0800									
0900									
1000									
1100									
1200									
1300									
1400									
1500									
1600									
1700									
1800									
1900									
2000									
2100									
2200									
2300									
2400									
Total....................									

Grand Total.........

Grand Total.........

(Not Including Insensible Loss)

Plus

Balance.................................

Total Volume of Blood Infused...

Minus

Figure 3.1

2 What volume of Omnopon should you draw up in the syringe if stock available is 20 mg/ml?

3 Hyoscine is available in a one ml ampoule and the dose is equivalent to 0.4 mg/ml. What volume is required for her 400 mcg order?

4 At 08.00 an intravenous infusion of 1 L of Compound Sodium Lactate (Hartman's solution) is commenced. This is to drip at 60 drops/minute via a drip chamber which emits 20 drops per ml. What volume of fluid is this woman currently receiving?

5 If the infusion continues at this rate, at what time would you expect this bag to complete?

Mrs Ferris returns to the ward at 13.00. She has a morphine infusion via a volumetric pump in situ, which was commenced at 11.00. It contains 60 mg of morphine in 100 ml of fluid, and is scheduled to last 25 hours.

6 What is the concentration (in mg/ml) of this medicated solution?

7 How much morphine will Mrs Ferris receive every four hours?

8 At what rate (volume/hour) should her infusion pump be set?

9 The Hartman's solution completes at 13.30 and 1 L of 0.9% sodium chloride is commenced, to complete in eight hours. At what speed should you set the drops per minute?

An anticoagulant (Heparin) is commenced. 10 000 units are to be given each day at 12-hourly intervals.

10 a How many units of Heparin should be given for a single dose?
    b If the only stock available is 25 000 units/ml, what volume should be given per dose?

11 During the afternoon Mrs Ferris becomes nauseated and is dry retching. Prochlorperazine (Stemetil) 12.5 mg is ordered. If stock available is equivalent to 0.0125 g per one ml ampoule, what volume should you give her?

12 Despite the anti-emetic drug being repeated later in the evening Mrs Ferris continues to feel very nauseated. The morphine is implicated as the cause and is removed at 19.00. With reference

to this infusion, what volume will be recorded on the intake chart?

13 At midnight Mrs Ferris asked for pain relief and 75 mg of pethidine was ordered. If the stock available was 100 mg/2 ml, what volume should have been given?

14 When you arrive on the ward at 07.30 next morning and visit Mrs Ferris, bag number three of her intravenous fluid order is in progress. The 1 L of 5% dextrose, which commenced at 21.00 last night, is to run over a 12-hour period. You note that approximately 160 ml remain in the bag. Is the infusion on schedule?

15 Mrs Ferris may sit out of bed today. She asks for pain relief prior to getting up. She may have codeine Phosphate 45 mg, 4-hourly PRN. Stock available is 30 mg scored tablets. What should you give her?

16 At 10.05 bag number four of her intravenous infusion is commenced and is to drip at 15 drops per minute. How much fluid per hour will this person receive from this infusion order?

17 How long would you expect this bag to last?

18 On day three Mrs Ferris is tolerating oral fluids quite well and may drink freely. Her family has brought her some pure apple juice but she asks you to dilute it to a 4 to 1 solution with iced water. How much apple juice will you put in the jug, and how much water is required to be added to make up 0.5 L of solution?

Bag four of the intravenous fluid order has been sluggish. The night staff reported that it has been dripping at approximately 10 drops/minute since midnight and this continues to be the rate of flow when you check it. You are asked to remove the intravenous infusion at 10.00.

19 How much fluid should be charted on the intake column of her fluid balance chart for this day's infusion?

20 On day four Mrs Ferris asks for 'something for her bowels'. She may have 20 mg of Bisacodyl PR. Suppositories available are of 10 mg strength. What will you give her?

EXERCISE FOUR

Mrs Patricia Myers is a 30-year-old woman who has been admitted to the ward with Pyelonephritis. On admission she is nauseous and is vomiting. She has pyrexia, dysuria with cloudy, foul-smelling urine and acute flank pain. She is an insulin dependent diabetic and is seven months pregnant. At 09.00 an intravenous line is inserted and she is to receive 3 L of intravenous fluid over the next 24 hours.

1   How many ml/hour should she receive from the above order?

2   If the drop factor for the giving set is 20 drops/ml, how fast should this infusion drip?

3   Intravenous pethidine, 60 mg, has been ordered 4-hourly PRN for pain relief. If available stock is 100 mg/2 ml, what volume should be drawn up?

4   The pethidine is to be given over a 4-minute period. How many mg/minute should she receive?

Intravenous metoclopramide hydrochloride (Maxolon) has been ordered for her vomiting. She may have a maximum of 0.5 mg/kg of body weight/day, to be given 4-hourly PRN.

5   Calculate the maximum daily dose of Maxolon that Mrs Myers may have if her weight is 60 kg.

6   From available stock of 10 mg/2 ml, calculate the volume to be drawn up for her initial dose of this medication.

Her insulin is due to be administered. She is to have 10 units of Actrapid and 25 units of Monotard (long-acting) insulin.

7   Which of the above is the 'clear' insulin?

8   Which insulin should be drawn up into the syringe first?

9   On the syringe in the diagram below, indicate the volume of each insulin amount that should be drawn up for this order.

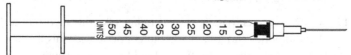

An intravenous antibiotic has been ordered. Mrs Myers is to have 2 grams of aztreonam (Azactam) every six hours for 48 hours. This medication is to be added to a secondary line of 0.9% sodium chloride in 100 ml. Stock available is 2 g of powder in a 10 ml vial, and manufacturing instructions suggest that the powder be mixed with 3 ml of sterile water to form a solution.

10 **a** Taking into account that the 2 g of powder will displace 2 ml of fluid when reconstituted, what volume of fluid will be in the vial when the powder and fluid are mixed?

b What is the concentration, in mg/ml, of this medicated solution?

11 You explain to Mrs Myers that the registered nurse is about to administer the ordered antibiotic. She expresses concern about the general effects that this medication could have on her unborn infant. How should you respond to her?

12 She then asks you if this medication will discolour her unborn child's teeth. How should this issue be addressed?

13 At what speed should you drip this medicated solution if the drop factor is 20 drops/ml and it is to last for one hour?

14 Paracetamol 1 gram is ordered to help reduce her fever. Ward stock is 500 mg tablets. What should you give her?

15 2 grams/day of ascorbic acid of has been ordered to help to acidify her urine. If this medication is to be given BD, and tablets available are 500 mg each, how many should she be given per dose?

A urinary antiseptic medication is to be introduced. 4 grams of nalidixic acid (Negram) per day is to be given in four equally divided doses for two weeks.

16 From available stock of 500 mg scored tablets, calculate her first dose of this medication.

17 Mrs Myers says that she would rather take this medication than the antibiotics and asks if she can continue with this if necessary when she returns home. What should be your response?

At 12.30 Mrs Myers presses her buzzer and asks for something for the unbearable bladder spasms she is experiencing. An anti-spasmodic medication, intravenous hyocine butylbromide (Buscopan) is ordered.

18 From available stock of 20 mg/ml, what volume should be drawn up for a 15 mg dose?

19 Just prior to handover at 15.00, you check her intravenous infusion and note that 820 ml of fluid has already infused. Is this the amount that you would have expected to have infused from the bag which commenced at 09.00?

20 If not, what is the correct amount of fluid that you would expect to see remaining in the bag at 15.00?

EXERCISE FIVE

You are caring for Mr Hollis, an elderly gentleman who has been transferred to the ward following a Myocardial Infarction five days ago. Mr Hollis has a history of alcoholism and is currently confused and aggressive due to Wernicke–Korsakoff Syndrome.

1 At 07.00 he is to have 150 mg of aspirin to suppress platelet aggregation. If stock available is 0.3 g tablets, what should you give him?

Following his shower at 08.30, he tells you that he has chest pain. Sublingual glyceryl trinitrate has been ordered to improve cardiac perfusion. He may have 600 mcg PRN for chest pain.

2 If stock available is 0.6 mg scored tablets, what should you give him?

At 10.00 several medications are due and you have been asked to give them under the supervsion of a registered nurse. He is to have sub-cutaneous enoxaparin (Clexane) 60 mg BD, oral thiamine (Vitamin B_1) 100 mg daily, oral pericyazine (Neulactil) 2.5 mg TDS, and oral trandolapril (Gopten) 0.5 mg daily.

3 Enoxaprin, a thrombolytic medication which seeks to remove formed thrombi, is available as 60 mg/ml. What volume should be given?

4 Thiamine or Vitamin B_1 is necessary to reduce neurological disorders caused by his high intake of alcohol. If stock on hand is 0.1 g tablets, how many tablets should you give him?

5 Pericyazine is to help to reduce Mr Hollis's episodes of aggression. The only tablets currently available on the ward are double scored 10 mg ones. What should you give him?

6 Trandolapril helps to control hypertension by reducing peripheral resistance. Stock on hand is 500 mcg capsules. How many capsules should you give him?

When lunch is delivered, Mr Hollis refuses to eat. You gently try to encourage him but he knocks the plate out of your hand and shouts abuse at you. He is seen by a medical officer and is ordered intramuscular Haloperidol, 2 mg.

7 From available stock of 5 mg/ml, what volume should you draw up?

Mr Hollis rests quietly after the haloperidol injection but becomes agitated when disturbed for a drink at 14.00. Diazepam 10 mg is ordered.

8 Stock available is 5 mg tablets. How many tablets should you give him?

Mr Hollis continues to refuse to drink, so an intravenous line is inserted. He is to have 1500 ml over a 24-hour period while he is not taking oral fluids.

9 How much fluid should you put into the burette each hour?

10 If the drop factor for the giving set is 20 drops/ml, to what speed, in drops/minute, should you adjust the rate of flow?

Mrs Smithers is admitted to the ward with an infected leg ulcer. She has non-insulin dependent Diabetes, is overweight and tells you that she smokes twenty cigarettes each day.

11 She is ordered flucloxacillin sodium (Flopen) 250 mg 6-hourly.
Stock available is equivalent to 0.25 g per capsule. Calculate the
number of capsules she should receive/dose.

12 Prior to dressing her wound, she is ordered 60 mg of intramuscular pethidine. If stock available is 100 mg/2 ml, calculate the
volume of this medication she should be given.

13 When you measure her blood glucose reading at 10.00, you report
your findings of 28 mmol/L. Sliding scale insulin is ordered. She
is to have two units of insulin for every 5 mmol/L above a reading
of 8 mmol/L. Calculate the dose you should give her now and
indicate the volume to be given on the 0.5 ml syringe below.

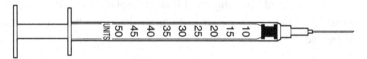

Mrs Smithers is seen by the dietician and is to commence a reducing
diet. She is to have a 6000 kilojoule diabetic diet.

14 She requires 45 g of protein per day. If 1 g of protein = 16 kj, what
percentage of her diet will be allocated to this nutrient?

15 She can have 15 g of fat in this diet. If 1 g of fat = 37 kj, what percentage of her diet is fat?

16 Carbohydrate is also 16 kj per gram. How many kilojoules will be
allocated for this food?

17 How many grams of carbohydrate will these kilojoules supply?

Next day when you return to duty, Mrs Smithers is flushed, dehydrated
and refusing to eat or drink fluids. Inspection of her wound suggests that
the infection is more aggressive than at first expected. An intravenous
infusion is established and intravenous antibiotics are commenced.

18 The 1 L of 0.9% sodium chloride is to infuse at the rate of
200 ml/hour for the first three hours. If the drop factor for the
giving set is 20 drops/ml, how fast should this infusion drip?

19 Intravenous flucloxacillin is increased to 0.5 g 6-hourly. Stock
available is 1 gram vials of powder which is to be reconstituted to

a strength of 100 mg/ml. What volume will need to be drawn up for her first dose?

20 The 0.5 g dose is to be added to 25 ml of intravenous fluid in the burette attached to the intravenous line and infused over a 10-minute period. How fast should this order drip to complete in the given time?

It is time to visit the Practical Nursing Calculations website again (see p. x) and complete the questions in Module Three, Assessment One. You have up to 30 minutes to complete this task and the use of a calculator to do this is discouraged.

For those of you who need further explanations of the scenarios covered to date, revise your learning at this point with the exercises provided.

EXERCISE SIX

You are caring for Mrs Peters who is recovering from a Cerebro-vascular Accident. She has a history of Diabetes and Hypertension.

1 A nasogastric tube is in situ and 1 L Osmolite (a nutrient) is dripping at 28 dpm. How long would you expect this bag to last if the drop factor for the giving set is 14 drops/ml?

2 Mrs Peters is to have frusemide, a diuretic, 40 mg each morning. Stock available for her use is a paediatric solution of 10 mg/ml. Calculate the volume to be given.

3 She is also to have 50 mg of captopril (Capoten) daily to treat her Hypertension, in two equally divided doses. Stock available is an oral solution of 5 mg/ml. Calculate the volume of a single dose of this medication.

4 The Capoten is to be mixed with water at a 1 (mg) in 10 (ml) ratio, before being introduced into the gastro-intestinal system via the nasogastric tube. How much water should you add to this medication to comply with the given instructions?

5 While she is ill, Mrs Peters, who is normally a non-insulin dependent diabetic, is to have 20 units of zinc suspension insulin BD. Stock available is 100 units per ml. On the diagram below, shade in the amount indicating what you will draw up for a single dose on this 0.5 ml syringe.

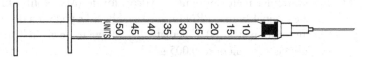

6 As Mrs Peters recovers, the nasogastric tube is removed. For the present she is to have 100 kilojoules per kg of ideal body weight per day. Her ideal body weight is 62 kg. How many kilojoules would this be?

7 a 20% of her nutrients are to come from fat. How many kilojoules will be allocated to this nutrient?
  b If 1 g of fat = 37 kilojoules, how many grams of fat will this diet include?

8 One week later, Mrs Peters is now mobile with assistance and may have an additional 20 kilojoules per kg of ideal body weight. What is her total kilojoule intake now?

Her blood glucose level has returned to normal and her insulin has now been discontinued. She is to have glibenclamide (Euglucon), a medication to help lower her blood glucose levels, 2.5 mg daily with her breakfast.

9 If stock available is 5 mg scored tablets, calculate the number of tablets she should be given.

10 She is now having captopril and frusemide in tablet form. With reference to Q 3 for her dose, calculate the number of tablets of captopril that she should be given for her morning dose if stock available is 12.5 mg tablets.

11 Frusemide is available in 40 mg tablets. How many tablets should she be given?

Mrs Betty Perkins has been admitted to the ward with right-sided abdominal pain for investigation. The pain is colicky in nature, and she is very nauseated. She also has a history of Hypertension and Angina. She weighs 60 kg. 100 mg of intramuscular pethidine has been ordered for her pain.

12 Stock available is 50 mg/ml. Calculate the volume to be given.

13 Intramuscular metoclopramide hydrochloride (Maxolon) 10 mg may be given 4-hourly PRN for nausea. She asks you for a dose of this medication at 11.00. Calculate the volume to be given if stock available is equivalent to 0.005 g/ml.

14 A provisional diagnosis of Biliary Colic is made and the anti-spasmodic medication, hyoscine butylbromide (Buscopan) 12 mg is to be given. Stock available is 20 mg/ml. Calculate the volume to be given.

15 Mrs Perkins begins to vomit. An intravenous line with 1 L of 0.9% sodium chloride is commenced. The fluid is to infuse over an 8-hour period and the drop factor for the giving set is 20 drops/ml. Calculate the rate of flow in drops/minute.

16 Next day, when you come on duty, Mrs Perkins is to be prepared for a Cholecystectomy. Her premedication is papaveretum (Omnopon) 15 mg and hyoscine 300 mcg. If stock available is a one ml ampoule containing 20 mg of Omnopon and 400 mcg of hyoscine, what volume should be drawn up?

17 On her return to the ward, a bag of Compound Sodium Lactate (Hartman's solution) is dripping at 60 drops/minute and 400 ml remain in the bag. How long will the remainder of this bag last?

18 7500 units of subcutaneous heparin is to be given. Stock available is 25 000 units/ml. Calculate the volume that should be drawn up.

Mrs Perkins develops tachycardia and is ordered a statim dose of intravenous Lanoxin, to slow and strengthen her heart beat. 10 mcg/kg of body weight to be given intravenously. The registered nurse asks you to work out the calculations.

19 a Lanoxin stock available is 0.5 mg/2 ml. Calculate the volume that should be given.

b It is to be added to 20 ml of fluid in the intravenous burette and given over a 20-minute period. Calculate the rate of flow, in drops/minute, for this medication.

20 She is to continue verapamil (Isoptin) 160 mg daily, to be given BD, which she has been taking for some time. If stock available is sugar-coated tablets of 40 mg, 80 mg or 160 mg, how many tablets and of what strength should you give her in a single dose?

EXERCISE SEVEN

You are to care for 18-year-old Julie who has been admitted to the ward for a Tonsillectomy in the morning. Julie is an epileptic whose condition is controlled by medication. She weighs 55 kg. She settles into the ward but tells you that she is very nervous about tomorrow's operation and is quite sure that she will 'not sleep a wink'. She is ordered nitrazepam 7.5 mg.

1 If stock available is 5 mg scored tablets, what should you give her?

She is to have phenytoin sodium (Dilantin) to control her seizures, 6 mg/kg of body weight/day, to be given TDS, morning, noon and nocte. From the total dose of this medication, she is to have 130 mg nocte.

2 **a** What is her total daily dose of this medication?
   b If stock available is 30 mg tablets, 50 mg chewable tablets and 100 mg capsules, what should you give her at bedtime?

Next morning when you come on duty, Julie has been allocated to you for her care. You visit her after handover and note that she has been fasting since midnight. You commence a fluid balance chart and organise her early morning dose of Dilantin which she may have with 50 ml of water.

3 Taking into account the stock available and using the given information above concerning the dose that is due, indicate how many tablets and of what strength she should be given.

At 08.30 her premedication of 60 mg of pethidine and 400 mcg of Atropine is due.

4 Pethidine is available as 100 mg/2 ml. Calculate the volume to be drawn up.

5 Atropine sulphate is available as 0.5 mg/ml. What volume should you draw up?

At 11.00 Julie returns to the ward with an intravenous infusion in progress. 640 ml of 5% dextrose remain in the 1 L bag and it is dripping at the rate of 60 drops per minute.

6 How long would you expect the remainder of the fluid to last if the drop factor for the giving set is 20 drops/ml and at what time should you expect it to complete?

At 11.30 Julie is quite distressed, she says her throat is extremely painful. She is ordered 60 mg of intravenous pethidine to be given over a 4-minute period.

7 From available stock (Q 4), calculate the volume to be drawn up.

8 How many mg should she receive every minute?

Half an hour later she vomits 600 ml of clotted blood. She is seen by a medical officer who orders a blood transfusion of 0.4 L, to be given as soon as possible.

9 If the normal blood volume for a person of Julie's size is 4 L, what percentage of her total blood volume has she just vomited?

10 At 12.15, prior to the commencement of the blood transfusion, you are asked to flush the intravenous line with 100 ml of 0.9% sodium chloride over a 30-minute period. State the purpose of this action and calculate the rate of flow in drops/minute.

400 ml of packed cells is commenced at 12.45. It is to infuse at the rate of 1 ml/minute for fifteen minutes.

11 To what rate of flow should you adjust the drops/minute and explain why the infusion rate is so slow.

At 13.10 you observe the registered nurse preparing to give Julie's midday dose of intravenous Dilantin. Remembering her usual oral dose (Q 2), she is to have only 75% of this dose because of the changed route of administration. Stock in the ward is 50 mg/ml.

12 Calculate the volume of this medication that should be drawn up.

13 At 14.00, Julie is permitted oral fluids of 30 ml of ice chips/hour. If she continues with this intake until 21.00 inclusive, how much oral fluid should be charted on the oral intake column of her fluid balance chart?

14 At 16.30 the blood transfusion completes and 1 L of 0.9% sodium chloride is commenced, to infuse over 8 hours. Calculate the rate of flow in drops per minute.

15 Julie's evening dose of Dilantin is also to be given intravenously. She is to have 0.1 gram of this medication. With reference to Q 11 for stock, what volume of medication would you expect to be given?

When you return to duty next morning, although feeling weak, Julie requests a shower and something to eat. She may have 14 mg of oral morphine prior to meals and at night, and you decide to give her some now, before her shower, so that her throat is more comfortable by the time her breakfast arrives.

16 Stock in the ward is a 200 ml bottle with a concentration of 2 mg/ml. How much mixture should you pour for her?

It is day three and Julie is up and about when you come on duty. Her nursing notes indicate that she is eating and drinking within normal limits. However, her haemoglobin (HB level) is lower than normal, so an iron supplement is to be given for four weeks. She is to have 20 ml of Fergon elixir (ferrous gluconate) per day, to be given BD. A Vitamin C supplement has been ordered to assist in the absorption of the iron.

17 If the dose is 60 mg of ferrous gluconate/ml, how much iron will she receive/dose?

18 Julie is to have 1 gram of vitamin C per day, to be given with the iron mixture. From available stock of 250 mg flavoured tablets, how many tablets should you give her at 18.00?

19 A friend brings Julie a 300 ml carton of orange juice but it burns her throat when she tries to swallow it. You offer to dilute it for her. How much water is required to make up a 3:1 solution?

20 Julie is ready for discharge and is told that she can have up to 3 grams of paracetamol each day for another week. How many 500 mg capsules will the pharmacist need to dispense to fulfil this order?

EXERCISE EIGHT

Mrs James has been admitted to the ward for abdominal surgery to remove an ovarian cyst. She has a six-week-old infant who is a boarder. Baby James is breast fed.

1 On the evening of her admission, Mrs James is ordered a sedative. She is to have phenobarbitone sodium (Nembutal) 100 mg. Stock in the ward is 50 mg capsules. How many should she be given?

Baby James is upset and you are nursing him. As part of your conversation with Mrs James, you ask her his weight. She tells you that he weighs 9 pounds 14 ounces and his length is 21.5 inches. You are aware that there are 16 ounces in one pound and 2.2 pounds in 1 kg.

2 Convert his weight to the metric measurement.

3 How many cm long is he if 1 inch equals 2.54 cm?

At 08.00 on the day of her operation, Mrs James's premedication is due. She is to have 12 mg of morphine and 0.5 mg of Atropine.

4 Calculate the volume of morphine that should be drawn up if stock available is 15 mg/ml.

5 Atropine is available as 600 mcg/ml. What volume is required?

While Mrs James is in the operating theatre, you are caring for baby James. His mother has left a jug of expressed breast milk in the refrigerator. At 10.15 he is fretful so you decide to feed him. You are aware that an infant of his age requires 460 kilojoules/kg of body weight/day.

6 What is his total daily kilojoule requirement?

7 a How many kj per feed would he need if he had six feeds per day?

  b If breast milk contains approximately 280 kilojoules/100 ml, how many ml would you expect him to drink now?

At 12.30, Mrs James returns to the ward. She has an intravenous infusion of Compound Sodium Lactate (Hartman's solution) dripping at 40 drops/minute. The drop factor for the giving set is 20 drops/ml.

8 How many ml/hour is Mrs James currently receiving?

9 If this bag commenced at 08.30 and 520 ml remain in the bag, at what time would you expect it to complete?

You are to observe the two registered nurses commencing a morphine infusion which will give Mrs James pain relief for the next 20 hours. She is to have 45 mg of morphine in a total of 30 ml of fluid.

10 If morphine is available as 15 mg/ml, what volume of this solution will be sterile normal saline?

11 How many milligrams of morphine will Mrs James receive every four hours?

12 What volume of fluid will the syringe pump deliver every hour?

13 Mrs James is to have 7500 units of Heparin (Calciparine) 12-hourly. If stock in the ward is 5000 units/0.2 ml, what volume should be drawn up?

14 Mrs James tells you that she is nauseous. She is ordered intramuscular prochlorperazine maleate (Stemetil) 10 mg. Stock on hand is 12.5 mg/ml. What volume should she be given?

15 The second bag of intravenous fluid is commenced. 1 L of 0.9% sodium chloride is to last for ten hours. How many ml/hour should be infused and how many drops/minute will fulfil the above order?

One of your tasks today is to make up the sodium hypochlorite (Milton) solution to sterilise baby James's bottles. You are to make up 4 L of solution.

16 a How much solute (Miltons) is required for a concentration of 1 in 80?
    b How much water will complete the job?

It is day two post-operatively and you are caring for Mrs James again. She has been assessed and bowel sounds are now present so you have been asked to encourage fluids. She has a 600 ml tin of mango and orange juice but is refusing to drink it because it is too sweet. She asks you to dilute it.

17 Make up a 1 L jug of fluid using the 600 ml of juice and 400 ml of ice water, and state the ratio in its most elementary form as _____ to_____.

18 Intravenous pain relief has now ceased and Mrs James may have 45 mg of codeine phosphate every six hours PRN. She asks for pain relief, so how many tablets should you give her if stock on hand is 30 mg tablets?

It is day four and Mrs James is being prepared for discharge. Because of the constipating effect of the codeine tablets, Metamucil has been ordered. Pharmacy has supplied her with a 100 gram tin of Metamucil and a box of 24 Panadeine tablets. She is concerned that this might not be enough, saying she won't feel like shopping for at least a week.

19 a If she is to take 14 grams (or 2 teaspoons) of Metamucil each day, will this tin last one week?

b What instructions should she be given with regards to taking the Metamucil for the most effective outcome of this medication?

20 Because the Panadeine also contains codeine, she has been asked to try to limit the intake of these tablets to no more than three each day. How long should this box of tablets last?

EXERCISE NINE

Bobby Jones is a young man who has recently returned from an overseas holiday. He has been admitted to hospital with severe diarrhoea and dehydration. He tells you that his normal weight is 65 kg. You are aware that he has lost 4.6 kg in the last two days.

1 State the approximate volume of fluid that he has lost.

2 Calculate the % of body weight lost.

An intravenous infusion is established and he is to have 4 L over the next 24 hours. The drop factor for the giving set is 20 drops/ml.

3 The first 1 L of 0.9% sodium chloride is to infuse in four hours. How many ml/hour should be delivered, and how fast should this infusion drip?

4 Bobby has a 0.5 L bottle of Kaomagma and may have 15 ml of mixture after each loose bowel action, to a maximum of 90 ml/day. How long could you expect this bottle to last?

Nausea is also a problem for Bobby. He has been ordered 7.5 mg of intravenous metoclopramide hydrochloride (Maxolon), 4-hourly PRN. Stock available is 10 mg/2 ml.

5 What volume of this medication should be drawn up for his ordered dose?

6 This medication is to be infused slowly. Taking into account the initial dose and the need for the remainder to go over a 2-minute period, how many mg/minute should you deliver?

You have been asked to go to lunch but you are keen to commence the second bag of intravenous fluid when the first one completes. You note that 130 ml remain in the bag and it is dripping at the rate of 82 drops per minute.

7 Have you time for a 30-minute lunch break?

8 The second bag is to infuse over a 5-hour period. State how many ml/hour will be delivered, and calculate the rate of flow in drops/minute?

It is day two and Bobby's diarrhoea continues. His weight has dropped a further 0.6 kg. He is to have intravenous ampicillin 3 grams/day, in four evenly divided doses. Ampicillin is available as 1 gram of powder in a 10 ml vial and manufacturing instructions indicate that it will displace 0.7 ml of fluid when reconstituted.

9 How much sterile water is required for a concentration of 100 mg/ml?

10 What is the total volume of the solution in the vial following reconstitution?

11 What volume should be drawn up for his first dose?

12 This medicated solution that has just been drawn up is to be added to the 20 ml of saline in the burette and delivered over a 15-minute period. How fast should it drip?

13 Bobby's condition stabilises following commencement of diphenoxylate hydrochloride (Lomotil) 30 mg/day, given 4-hourly. How many mg/dose should he receive?

14 Lomotil is available as 2.5 mg tablets. How many tablets should he be given per dose?

When you come on duty next morning, Bobby tells you that he is much better, his diarrhoea has decreased considerably and he can now retain oral fluids. He is permitted diluted apple juice.

15 How much iced water is required to make up 500 ml of diluted apple juice if the ratio he is permitted is 3 to 2?

16 His intravenous infusion has now been reduced to 50 ml/hour. How many drops/minute will deliver this order?

17 How long will his 500 ml bag last?

18 If the infusion was commenced at 08.00, when would you expect it to complete?

19 The Lomotil has been reduced to 5 mg/day, to be given in two equally divided doses. How many tablets (dose in Q 14) should you give him for his morning dose?

Day four and Bobby can go home when his present bag of intravenous fluid completes. He asks you how long he needs to remain as he wants to let his girlfriend know when to collect him.

20 If 40 ml remain and this is dripping at 15 drops/minute, how long will it last?

EXERCISE TEN

Mrs Jenner has been admitted to the ward for a Haemorrhoidectomy in the morning. She has been allocated to your care. At 22.00 she is still awake and is quite restless, and says that she is worrying about her operation in the morning.

1 Nitrazepam 10 mg has been ordered to help her to relax and get to sleep. Stock in the ward is equivalent to 0.005 g/tablet. What should you give her?

At 07.30 next morning when you complete handover, her premedication is due. As this lady has been allocated to you for care, you are to give this medication. She has been ordered 80 mg of pethidine and 300 mcg of Hyocine.

2 If the pethidine stock available is 100 mg/2 ml, what volume should you draw up?

3 Hyocine stock is 0.4 mg/ml. What volume should you draw up?

Mrs Jenner returns to the ward at 10.45 and has an intravenous line in situ, with a drop factor of 20 drops/ml. 270 ml remain in the bag and it is dripping at 60 drops per minute.

4 How many ml/minute is she receiving from this infusion?

5 How long would you expect the remainder of the fluid to last?

A pethidine infusion was established in Recovery. Mrs Jenner is to receive 300 mg of pethidine over a 25-hour period. The pethidine has been added to a 100 ml bag of 0.9% sodium chloride and is being delivered via a volumetric pump connected as a secondary line on her main infusion.

6 What is the concentration (in mg/ml) of this medicated solution?

7 To what speed (in ml/hour) should the infusion pump be set?

8 How many mg of pethidine is Mrs Jenner receiving every four hours?

9 Is this within normal limits for an adult weighing 65 kg?

Mrs Jenner's bag of 0.9% sodium chloride completes and 1 L of 5% dextrose is commenced. This bag of fluid is to infuse at 40 drops/minute for the first four hours and then 30 drops per minute for the remainder of the bag.

10 How many ml/hour will you need to put into the burette each hour for the first four hours?

11 How many ml/hour will need to be run into the burette for the remainder of the fluid?

12 How long would you expect this bag to last?

Mrs Jenner rings her bell to ask for assistance to get onto the commode to pass urine. When you help her back to bed, she tells you that her pain is unbearable. An order is made to give her a bolus dose of 12 mg of pethidine over a four-minute period.

13 How many mg per minute should she receive from this order?

14 How many ml per minute will contain the ordered dose?

15 To what speed (ml/hr) should the pump be adjusted to deliver the 12 mg in four minutes?

16 Oral fluids are commenced and Mrs Jenner is advised to have approximately 100 ml per hour for the next four hours, but when you visit her two hours later, you note 0.2 L remaining in her 1 L jug. What volume should be charted on the oral intake column of her fluid balance chart?

17 Mrs Jenner complains of nausea. Oral metoclopramide hydrochloride (Maxolon) 5 mg is ordered. If stock on hand is 10 mg tablets, what should she be given?

18 Mrs Jenner rings her bell to tell you she has vomited her tablet. She is now ordered 7.5 mg of intramuscular Maxolon. Stock in the ward is 10 mg/2 ml. What volume should be drawn up for this statim dose?

19 Next morning when you return to duty, you continue to care for Mrs Jenner. You check her intravenous infusion and note it is dripping at 20 drops per minute. What volume of fluid is she receiving each hour from this order?

20 The infusion can be removed on completion of the present bag. Mrs Jenner tells you she will shower when the line is removed. How long will she have to wait for her shower if 90 ml remain in the bag?

It is time to visit the Practical Nursing Calculations website (see p. x) again and complete Module Three, Assessment Two. You should be able to complete this in less than 30 minutes and gain a 100% pass, without the use of your calculator.

 # ANSWERS

EXERCISE ONE

1 **a** 60 ml/hr **b** 60 ml/hr **c** 72 ml/hr **d** 36 ml/hr

2 **a** 40 ml/hr **b** 30 ml/hr **c** 40 ml/hr **d** 20 ml/hr

3 **a** 50 ml/hr **b** 60 ml/h **c** 30ml/hr **d** 25 ml/hr

4 **a** 120 ml/hr **b** 90 ml/hr **c** 60 ml/hr **d** 120 ml/hr

5 **a** 60 ml/hr **b** 30 ml/hr **c** 80 ml/hr **d** 100 ml/hr

6 2 tablets

7 1 tablet

8 Potassium chloride

9 Some diuretic medications cause potassium to be excreted in the urine, therefore this is a replacement.

10 It should be explained that these tablets should not be crushed as they are enteric coated to allow for a slow release of potassium in the intestines.

11 1/2 tablet

12 200 ml

13 600 mcg

14 2 tablets

15 1 × 20 mg tablet

16 2 tablets

17 Salicylates potentiate the action of tolbutamide.

18 0.45 g or 450 mg

19 500 mg/dose

20 2 capsules/dose

EXERCISE TWO

1 2 tablets

2 1.2 ml

3 0.5 ml

4 **a** 2 ml/minute **b** 120 ml/hour

5 At 16.20

6 **a** 6 ml **b** 6 ml

7 3 mg/ml

8 12 mg/hour

9 4 ml/hour

10 3 mg/minute

11 1 ml/minute

12 60 ml/hour for four minutes only

13 It should complete at 12.00 rather than 13.00 tomorrow.

14 **a** 100 ml/hour **b** 33 drops/minute

15 28 drops/minute

16 Yes, it is close to running to schedule. 583 ml should be in the bag.

17 400 ml

18 48 ml

19 See fluid balance chart (Fig. 3.5)

20 12 tablets

EXERCISE THREE

1 1 tablet

2 0.8 ml

3 1 ml

	FLINDERS MEDICAL CENTRE **FLUID BALANCE CHART**			Ward		
				Surname	SMART	
				Other Names	Monique Helen	
				D.O.B./Sex	6 – 7 - 1987 female	
Medical Officer:		Date:		Address		
				Medi. No.	567 891 234	

	INTAKE				OUTPUT					
Time	By Mouth or Tube (Description)	ml	Intravenous	ml	Vomitus or Aspirate	ml	Faeces and Other Drainage (Description)	ml	Urine ml	
0100			4% D in 0.18%N/s 8/F (233)	4 100						
0200				4 100						
0300			0.9% Sod. Chl. (1000)	4 33+50						
0400				4 83						
0500				4 83						
0600				4 83						
0700				4 83						
0800				4 83						
0900				4 83						
1000	Ice chips (40)			4 83						
1100	(40)	40		4 83						
1200	(40)	40		4 83						
1300	(40)	40		83						
1400	(40)	40		83						
1500	(40)	40		37						
1600	(40)	40								
1700	(40)	40								
1800	(40)	40								
1900	(40)	40								
2000	(40)	40								
2100		40								
2200										
2300										
2400										
Total		440		1281						
Grand Total			1721				Grand Total			

(Not Including Insensible Loss)

Plus
Balance.....................................
Minus

Total Volume of
Blood Infused...

Figure 3.5

4 180 ml/hour

5 At approximately 13.30

6 0.6 mg/ml

7 9.6 mg

8 4 ml/hour

9 42 drops/minute

10 **a** 5000 units/dose   **b** 0.2 ml/dose

11 1 ml

12 32 ml

13 1.5 ml

14 Slightly slower than schedule, 125 ml should remain at 07.30

15 $1\frac{1}{2}$ tablets

16 45 ml/hour

17 Approximately 22 hours and 15 minutes

18 400 ml apple juice and 100 ml water

19 300 ml

20 2 suppositories

EXERCISE FOUR

1 125 ml/hour

2 42 drops/minute

3 1.2 ml

4 15 mg/minute

5 30 mg

6 1 ml (30 ÷ 6 doses)

7 Actrapid

8 The clear insulin

9 35 units in total, as below

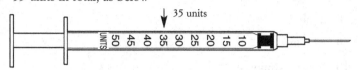

35 units

10 a 5 ml   **b** 400 mg/ml

11 Although this medication crosses the placental barrier, there has been no evidence of mutagenic changes to the foetus in laboratory studies (MIMS 2001).

12 While studies are limited, there is no evidence of any abnormalities from this drug.

13 35 drops/minute

14 2 tablets

15 2 tablets

16 2 tablets

17 This medication should be used with caution in the third trimester of pregnancy, so it is suggested that it should be discontinued well before delivery date.

18 0.75 ml

19 No, it is infusing too fast, 750 ml should have infused.

20 250 ml

EXERCISE FIVE

1 1/2 tablet

2 1 tablet

3 1 ml

4 1 tablet

5 1/4 tablet

6 1 capsule

7   0.4 ml

8   2 tablets

9   62.5 ml

10   21 drops/minute

11   1 capsule/dose

12   1.2 ml

13   8 units or 0.08 ml, as below

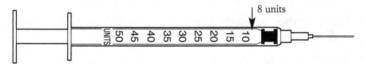

14   12% is protein

15   9.25% is fat

16   4725 kilojoules

17   295.3 grams

18   67 drops/minute

19   5 ml/dose

20   60 drops/minute

EXERCISE SIX

1   8 hours 20 minutes

2   4 ml

3   5 ml

4   245 ml

5   0.2 ml or 20 units, as below

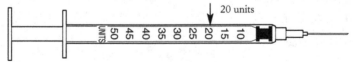

6 6200 kilojoules

7 **a** 1240 kj   **b** 33.5 grams of fat

8 7440 kilojoules

9 1/2 tablet

10 2 tablets

11 1 tablet

12 2 ml

13 2 ml

14 0.6 ml

15 42 drops/minute

16 0.75 ml

17 2 hours 13 minutes

18 0.3 ml

19 a 2.4 ml   **b** 22 drops/minute

20 1 × 80 mg tablet

EXERCISE SEVEN

1 $1\frac{1}{2}$ tablets

2 **a** 330 mg   **b** 1 × 100 mg and 1 × 30 mg tablet

3 1 × 100 mg capsule

4 1.2 ml

5 0.8 ml

6 3 hours 33 minutes, to complete at 14.30

7 1.2 ml

8 15 mg/minute

9 15% of her blood

10 dextrose can cause platelet aggregation so the line should contain 0.9% sodium chloride to prevent haemolysis, or breakdown of red blood cells (Crisp & Taylor 2001). This solution should drip at 67 drops/minute.

11 20 drops/minute. If the introductory rate of flow is slow, early detection of a transfusion reaction reduces possible harmful consequences.

12 1.5 ml

13 240 ml (30 ml × 8 hours)

14 42 drops/minute

15 2 ml

16 7 ml

17 600 mg/dose

18 2 tablets

19 100 ml

20 42 × 500 mg capsules

EXERCISE EIGHT

1 2 capsules

2 4.5 kg (approximately)

3 54.6 cm

4 0.8 ml

5 0.8 ml

6 2070 kilojoules

7 **a** 345 kj/feed **b** 123 ml/feed

8 120 ml/hour

9 16.50

10 27 ml (30 ml – 3 ml morphine)

11 9 mg/4 hours

12 1.5 ml

13 0.3 ml

14 0.8 ml

15 100 ml/hour, 33 drops/minute

16 **a** 50 ml   **b** 3950 ml

17 3 to 2

18 $1\frac{1}{2}$ tablets

19 **a** Yes, (100 g ÷ 14 g)   **b** Drink 250 ml with the medication, repeat fluid

20 8 days

EXERCISE NINE

1 4.6 L

2 Approximately 7%

3 250 ml/hour, 83 drops/minute

4 $5\frac{1}{2}$ days

5 1.5 ml

6 2.5 mg/minute initially, then 2.5 mg or 0.5 ml after one and two minutes

7 Only just! It should last just over 32 minutes.

8 200 ml/hour and 67 drops/minute

9 9.3 ml

10 10 ml

11 7.5 ml

12 36–37 drops/minute

13 5 mg/dose

14 2 tablets/dose

15 200 ml of iced water

16 Approximately 17 drops/minute

17 10 hours

18 At 18.00

19 1 tablet/dose

20 Approximately 53 minutes

EXERCISE TEN

1 2 tablets

2 1.6 ml

3 0.75 ml

4 3 ml/minute

5 90 minutes or $1\frac{1}{2}$ hours

6 3 mg/ml

7 4 ml/hour

8 48 mg/4 hours

9 Yes

10 120 ml/hour

11 90 ml/hour

12 9 hours 46 minutes

13 3 mg/minute

14 1 ml of fluid

15 60 ml/hour

16 800 ml

17 1/2 tablet

18 1.5 ml

19 60 ml/hour

20 $1\frac{1}{2}$ hours

4

Paediatric Dosages

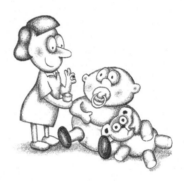

Objectives

After completing the given calculations, it is expected that you should be able to calculate safe dosages and administer medications to a child, and include in this:

1 identifying the steps required to determine body surface area using a nomogram (paediatric or adult)

2 calculating dosages per kilogram of body weight

3 administering parenteral paediatric medications, including those which involve reconstitution

4 verifying safe dosages using a comparison with recommended paediatric dosages

5 understanding the theoretical management of an intravenous infusion, embracing daily fluid needs

6 being familiar with using volumetric pumps, encompassing the administration of bolus doses

EXERCISE ONE

MEDICATION DOSAGES FOR CHILDREN

When medications are being considered for children, it is important to remember that children are not small adults and many factors need to be taken into account when calculating a dose. Factors that need to be considered include age, weight, size, physiological and psychological state, and the fact that many organ systems are yet to reach maturity. In most cases, drug dosages are worked out according to a child's weight, but the child's body surface area is considered to give a more precise evaluation. In most instances, the recommended paediatric dose has been calculated by the manufacturers, but this is not always the case.

It is not your role as a student to independently determine a medication dosage for a child. However, formulas and exercises are provided to demonstrate to you how a dosage could be established should there be an emergency for you when checking a dose.

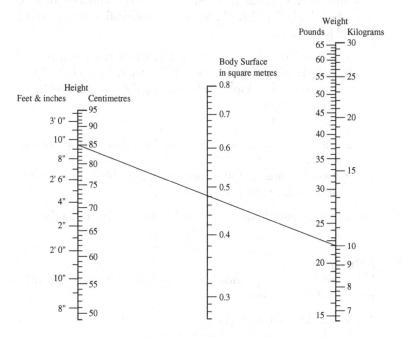

Figure 3.1 *A nomogram (Du Bois 1936)*

Many pharmacological textbooks offer formulas to calculate medication dosages but for the purpose of the following exercises, only weight and body surface areas will be used. Illustrated in Fig. 3.1 is a nomogram which is used to calculate a body surface area by finding the child's height and weight on the scale and then joining the two with a straight line. The point where the line crosses the surface area will indicate that child's body surface area (BSA).

The example given demonstrates how to find the BSA of a child who is 85 cm in height and weighs 10 kg. You will note that the line crosses the surface area point at 0.48 metres squared (m²). If the measurements are not within the nomogram of the child, then refer to the nomogram of the adult using the same principle to determine the BSA.

Example

Christine is 14 kg and 94 cm tall. She has been ordered drug X, 1 gram per square metre (m²) of body surface area (BSA) per day, to be given 6-hourly. Stock available is a mixture with a concentration of 25 mg per ml of fluid. Calculate the volume of medication that should be poured for each dose.

   a Determine her BSA using the nomogram. It is 0.6 m².
   b Calculate her daily dose of drug X by converting her BSA to a fraction and multiply the fraction by the ordered dose (in mg)

$$\frac{60}{100} \times \frac{1000}{1} = 600 \text{ mg}$$

   c Find the number of mg per dose by dividing 600 by 4, which is 150 mg/dose.
   d Dose required is 150 mg and stock available is 25 mg per ml, so the dose to be poured is 6.0 ml.

Please note, some children will need to be assessed using the adult nomogram.

Activity

Using the nomogram provided in the appendix, find the body surface areas in m² for the following

1   **a** a child weighing 15 kg who is 100 cm tall
   b a baby who is 55 cm long and weighs 4 kg
   c a teenager 160 cm tall and weighs 35 kg

2 **a** a child who is 102 cm tall and weighs 16 kg
   b a man who is 192 cm tall and weighs 72 kg
   c a toddler who is 72 cm tall and weighs 11.5 kg

3 **a** a teenager who is 154 cm tall and weighs 30 kg
   b a child who is 90 cm tall and weighs 25 kg
   c a baby who is 36 cm long and weighs 1.2 kg

Jamie, aged three months, is to have 100 mg of drug A per m^2 of body surface area per day. Jamie is 56 cm long and weighs 5.2 kg.

4 **a** What is his body surface area in m^2?
   b Calculate the dose of medication required.
   c Jamie's medication is to be given 6-hourly. How many mg should he have per dose?
   d Drug A is available as a mixture with a concentration of 5 mg/ml. What volume should be measured (in a syringe) for Jamie's midday dose?

Ten-year-old Sally is to have 200 mg of drug B per m^2 of body surface area per day. Sally is 130 cm tall and weighs 28 kg.

5 **a** What is Sally's body surface area in m^2?
   b How much medication (in mg) should Sally have each day?
   c Sally's medication is to be given 6-hourly, and it is available as a mixture with a concentration of 0.01 g per ml. How much medicine should you measure for her 10.00 dose?

Two-year-old Edward has a malignancy. He is to have 1 g of drug C per m^2 of body surface area per day. He weighs 9 kg and his height is 66 cm.

6 **a** How many mg of drug C should Edward have each day?
   b Edward's medication is to be given BD and stock available is a mixture with a concentration of 20 mg/ml. How much medication should you pour for him for his 18.00 dose?

7 Christine, who is 8 years old and weighs 17 kg, is 102 cm tall. She is to have 1.4 g of drug D per m^2 of body surface area. This medication is to be given 6-hourly and is available as an injection with a concentration of 500 mg/ml. Calculate the volume to be given/dose.

You are caring for six-year-old Connie who has severe Tonsillitis and Otitis Media. She has a fever and is very fretful. Connie has been ordered amoxycillin syrup, 20 mg/kg/day, to be given 8-hourly.

8 a If Connie weighs 24 kg, what is her daily dose of this medication?

    b From available stock of 125 mg/5 ml, what volume should you pour for her 10.00 dose?

9 Connie is to have paracetamol elixir, 10 ml every four hours for her sore throat and to help to reduce her fever. She is to have this mixture diluted with water at a 1 to 1 ratio. What is the total volume of fluid per dose?

10 If the paracetamol mixture available is 24 mg/ml, how much actual paracetamol should Connie receive per dose?

11 If the recommended dose is 15 mg/kg, is this a suitable dose for a child of Connie's age and weight? If not, what dose should she be given?

12 Connie is to have a 1 in 10 Cepacaine gargle for her throat. State the volume of water required to make a 100 ml gargle.

Connie complains that she is itchy. Your assessment of Connie shows that she has an urticarial rash extending over a large area of her trunk. The medical officer is notified and suspends the amoxycillin.

13 Connie is ordered the antihistamine promethazine HCl (Phenergan) elixir 30 mg/day to be given in three equally divided doses. Stock available is a 100 ml bottle with a concentration of 5 mg/5 ml. Calculate the volume of medicine she should receive each dose.

Following the suspension of Connie's amoxycillin, her temperature rises to 40.2°C. She is ordered cefaclor monohydrate (Ceclor) suspension 6-hourly.

14 a A statim dose of 0.25 g is to be given. If stock available is 125 mg/5 ml, what volume should be poured for this dose?

    b Remembering that Connie's amoxycillin was suspended due to a probable allergic reaction to penicillin, should you question this medication order? Explain your answer.

15 Connie's condition does not improve. An intravenous line is inserted and 1 L of 5% dextrose is commenced. This intravenous fluid is infusing via a micro-dropper at 60 drops/minute. How long would you expect this flask to last?

Intravenous erythromycin, 40 mg/kg/day, is to be given in four equally divided doses. You are assisting the registered nurse to give this medication. Stock available is a 10 ml vial containing 1 gram of medicated powder. Instructions accompanying this medication tell you to add 9 ml of sterile water for a concentration of 100 mg/ml.

16 **a** What is the daily dose of this medication for Connie?
  b How many mg should she receive for a single dose?
  c How many ml will be in the vial when the powder and water are reconstituted (mixed)?
  d What volume should be drawn up for a single dose of this medication for Connie?

17 **a** Connie is to have 0.5% chloramphenicol (Chloromycetin) ear drops. If each ml of fluid in the bottle contains 20 potential drops, how many drops of chloramphenicol are there in a 10 ml bottle?
  b If Connie is to have four drops in her right ear, four times each day, how long will this bottle last?

When you return to duty next morning, Connie is looking much more cheerful. Her first bag of intravenous fluid (5% dextrose) is dripping at 70 drops per minute and 90 ml remain. Her next bag of fluid is to be 500 ml of 0.9% sodium chloride.

18 **a** Have you time to bath another child (about 30 minutes) before the dextrose solution completes?
  b If the 0.9% sodium chloride is to last for ten hours, how fast should it drip?

19 Connie asks for some orange juice to drink. The registered nurse asks you to dilute it to a 4 to 1 ratio. How much orange juice to water is required to make up a 200 ml glass?

20 Connie's intravenous erythromycin has been changed to an oral suspension. Stock available is 125 mg/5 ml. Calculate the volume you should measure for a single dose, equivalent to the intravenous dose.

EXERCISE TWO

You are on a late shift and you have been asked to care for Karen who has just been admitted to the ward for an Appendicectomy in the morning. Karen is 12 years old and weighs 40 kg.

1   At 22.00 Karen rings her buzzer and tells you she cannot get to sleep. She is ordered nitrazepam 7.5 mg. Stock available in the ward is 5 mg scored tablets. How many tablets should she be given?

When you come on duty next morning, you are to follow through with your care of Karen. On visiting her after handover, you note that her premedication is due at 07.45. She is to have 20 mg of promethazine hydrochloride (Phenergan) elixir to make her drowsy prior to her operation.

2   Stock available on the ward is an elixir containing 5 mg/5 ml. How much medication should you pour for Karen?

At 10.30 Karen returns to the ward from Recovery and you are completing the routine observations required to be carried out when a client returns to the ward following surgery. An intravenous infusion is in place and the fluid order sheet indicates that the 1 L of 4% dextrose in 0.18 % sodium chloride is to last for eight hours.

3   How many ml/hour should Karen receive from this infusion, and if the drop factor for the giving set is 20 drops/ml, how many drops/minute would you expect to see infusing?

4   If this bag was commenced at 08.30, when would you expect it to complete? If 750 ml remain in the bag, is this infusion running to schedule?

A medicated infusion is to be established to help to control Karen's pain. She is to have 200 mg of pethidine in 100 ml of 0.9% sodium chloride. This solution is to be delivered via a volumetric pump and is connected as a 'secondary' line to her main infusion, which is gravity controlled with a macro giving set. The medicated infusion is to last for 25 hours. The registered nurses ask you to check their calculations.

5 If the usual dose of pethidine for a child of Karen's age and weight is 1.5 mg/kg every four hours, is the ordered dose within normal limits?

6 If injectable pethidine is available as 50 mg/ml, what volume will need to be drawn up for this task?

7 What is the concentration, in mg/ml, of this medicated infusion?

8 How many ml/hour will deliver the ordered dose of medication?

Karen's appendix was very inflamed and so an intravenous antibiotic (Amoxil) is prescribed. She is to have amoxycillin sodium 0.5 g every six hours. The registered nurse asks you to prepare the antibiotic under her supervision. Stock to be used is a 10 ml vial containing 1 gram of amoxycillin powder. Accompanying instructions indicate that the powder will displace 0.7 ml of fluid when reconstitution occurs.

9 What volume of sterile water for injection is required to reconstitute this medication to a concentration of 100 mg/ml?

10 What volume of medication should be drawn up for her first dose?

This antibiotic will require further dilution because if the dose is too concentrated it will irritate the child's vein. For this reason, it is to be added to 45 ml of intravenous fluid in the burette.

11 a What is the concentration of this medication solution (in mg/ml) when it is added to the fluid in the burette?
   b How many drops per minute will deliver this solution over a 20-minute period?

At 12.30 Karen calls you to tell you that she 'feels sick'. She has an order for metoclopramide hydrochloride (Maxolon) 3 mg, to be given by slow intravenous injection.

12 From available stock of 10 mg/2 ml, what volume should be drawn up for this order?

Despite the anti-emetic, Karen begins to dry retch. She is very distressed and says her pain is unbearable. A bolus dose of pethidine, 10 mg, is ordered to be delivered over a 4-minute period.

13 a How many mg/minute should she receive from this bolus dose?

b What volume of solution will deliver the calculated dose (mg)/minute?

14 To what speed, in ml/hour, should the pump be adjusted to comply with the bolus dose order?

Because Karen begins to vomit, her intravenous fluid intake is continued. Her second bag of intravenous fluid, which is 1 L of 5% dextrose, commenced at 16.40 and is to last for ten hours.

15 How many ml would you expect to be added to the burette every hour and how many drops per minute are required to deliver the above order?

When you return to duty at 07.00 the next morning, you continue with your care of Karen. At 07.30, you check her notes and see that flask number three is already well under way. The written order states that this 1 L bag of 0.9% sodium chloride is to last for twelve hours.

16 You check the rate of flow and note that it is 35 drops per minute. How many ml/hour would be delivered at this rate of flow? What is the correct rate of flow for this infusion?

Karen is permitted fluid today as bowel sounds are now present. She can have 30 ml of ice chips hourly for four hours and then clear fluids if she is tolerating the ice chips.

17 If she has five small tubs (30 ml) of ice, what volume of fluid will be recorded on the oral intake column of her fluid balance chart?

18 At 13.00 Karen asks you to make her half a jug of weak cordial. What volume of cordial is required for a 10% solution of 500 ml?

19 It is day three and Karen's intravenous infusion has been removed. She is to have her Amoxil orally. With reference to Q 9 for dose, how many 250 mg capsules should she be given for her 10.00 dose?

20 She asks for something for her pain. She is now permitted 750 mg of paracetamol four-hourly PRN. From available stock of 500 mg scored tablets, how many should she be given?

EXERCISE THREE

You are still in the Children's Ward and today you have been allocated to care for five-year-old Stella under the guidance of a registered nurse. Stella has been admitted to the ward with Cellulitis of her right leg following an injury to the leg. She weighs 20 kg, and on admission is febrile, dehydrated and very tearful. At 09.00 an intravenous line is established. Stella is to have 0.5 L of 0.9% sodium chloride over the next ten hours.

1 How much fluid should you run into the burette every hour, and if a micro-dropper is in use, how many drops per minute should she receive from this order?

Stella's leg is to be cleaned every four hours. As she sees you approaching with the dressing trolley she begins to scream. You check her medication orders and note that she may have pethidine, 0.75 mg/kg of body weight, four-hourly PRN for pain.

2 How many mg of pethidine should she have per dose?

3 What volume should you draw up if stock available is 50 mg/ml?

Stella is ordered Panadol elixir for her pyrexia. She is to have 10 ml 4-hourly PRN. On checking the medicine cabinet you discover two strengths of Panadol elixir, 24 mg/ml and 48 mg/ml.

4 How will you determine which mixture to use?

5 How many mg is in the dose you should give?

6 If the ideal dose for Stella is 15 mg/kg of body weight, have you chosen the correct medication?

Amoxycillin trihydrate is ordered to combat her infection. She is to have 25 mg/kg of body weight/day, to be given in four equally divided doses.

7 Calculate her daily dose of this medication.

8 How many mg should she receive for a single dose?

9 From available stock (Amoxil syrup) of 125 mg/5 ml, what volume of medicine should you pour for her first dose?

10 Vitamin C is ordered to promote healing of her leg. She is to have 1 g/day, to be given QID, for two weeks. What does the abbreviation QID mean?

11 From available stock of 0.5 g scored tablets, what should you give her at 10.00?

Stella's condition deteriorates as the day progresses. Her temperature continues to rise and she is refusing oral fluids because she says she feels sick. At 14.00 when the 0.5 L bag of 0.9% sodium chloride completes, 1 L of 5% dextrose is commenced.

12 If this bag of fluid is to infuse at the rate of 75 ml/hour, how long should it last?

13 The giving set is changed to one with a drop factor of 20, how fast should this fluid drip?

The amoxycillin (Amoxil) is to be given intravenously now. You are observing the registered nurse draw up this medication. You note that the dose has been increased to 40 mg/kg/day, to be given 6-hourly. The vial of 0.5 g of powder is to be reconstituted to a strength of 100 mg/ml. She asks you to work out the necessary calculations.

14 What has the daily dose of Amoxil been increased to?

15 How many mg/dose should Stella receive from the new order?

16 If the Amoxil powder in the vial displaces 0.4 ml of fluid when reconstituted, how much fluid needs to be added to the vial to achieve the desired concentration of 100 mg/ml?

17 What volume of medication would you expect the registered nurse to draw up for a single dose?

Meanwhile, Stella is ordered prochlorperazine (Stemetil) for her nausea. She may have a total of 15 mg/day, to be given TDS PRN. She has refused a tablet so a suppository is ordered, as it is less painful than a deep intramuscular injection.

18 Suppositories are available as 5mg/suppository. How many should be given for her first dose?

The registered nurse is about to give the intravenous Amoxil. She informs you that a concentration of no more than 5 mg/ml is to be infused over a 30-minute period.

19 If the drawn up dose is added to the 48 ml of fluid currently in the burette, has the minimum desired concentration been achieved?

20 How fast should this medicated infusion drip to deliver the ordered dose in the specified time?

EXERCISE FOUR

Four-year-old Billy has been admitted to the ward with Pneumonia. On admission he is febrile, dehydrated and tearful. His weight is 18 kg and height is 77 cm.

1 What is Billy's body surface area (BSA) in m^2?

2 Billy is to have a daily fluid intake of 2.5 L per m^2 of BSA. How much fluid per day will he have?

3 This fluid is to be administered via a volumetric pump. To what rate of flow, in ml/hour, will you need to adjust the pump?

Ampicillin sodium, 50 mg/kg/day, is to be given to combat his chest infection. This medication is to be given 4-hourly via his intravenous line.

4 What is his daily dose of this medication?

5 How many mg/dose should he receive?

6 The ampicillin is available in vials containing 250, 500 or 1000 mg of powdered medication. Which strength would be most practical to use for Billy's 10.00 dose considering that any unused portion will need to be discarded?

7 1 gram of this powder will displace 0.8 ml of fluid when reconstituted, so how much water will you need to add to your chosen vial strength, to achieve a concentration of 100 mg/ml?

8 What volume of medication will need to be drawn up for a single dose of this medication?

9 Billy is ordered salbutamol sulfate inhalations every four hours for his asthma. He is to have 0.02 ml/kg 4-hourly. How many ml/dose should he have?

10 This medication is to be given at a 1 to 2 ratio using normal saline as the solvent. What volume of saline is required for this task?

11 How much fluid (in total) should be added to the inhaler?

Theophylline (Elixophyllin elixir), 20 mg/kg/day, is to be given in four equally divided doses. Stock available in the ward is a 500 ml bottle containing 80 mg of theophylline/15 ml of mixture.

12 How many mg/day has he been ordered?

13 How many mg/dose should he receive?

14 How much mixture should you pour for his morning dose?

You are to encourage Billy to drink fluids as his temperature remains higher than expected. He is to be offered 50 ml of fluid every hour for the next six hours.

15 If Billy drinks half of what is offered, how much fluid should be charted on the oral intake column of his fluid balance chart?

16 Paracetamol (Panadol elixir), 10 ml, is also to be given to help to reduce his fever. Stock available is 24 mg/ml or 48 mg/ml. Calulate the total dose using both strengths.

17 Which strength should you use if the accepted dose for Billy is 15 mg/kg of body weight/dose?

Billy's condition does not improve. He remains febrile, fretful, and has a productive cough which is distressing to him. His oral fluid intake is poor. His intravenous infusion is increased to 0.1 L per hour for the next four hours to be delivered via the volumetric pump.

18 How many ml/hour will this new order deliver?

19 State the purpose of using a volumetric pump in preference to the micro-dropper for children.

20 a The intravenous ampicillin sodium is increased to 1.5 g/day, to be given 8-hourly. Calculate a single dose of this medication in mg.

b If the concentration of the medication is 100 mg/ml, what volume is required for a single dose?

EXERCISE FIVE

Seven-year-old Amy has been admitted to the ward with severe diarrhoea and vomiting. She is being nursed in a side room with additional precautions for enteric isolation. Her height is 105 cm and her weight is 24 kg. She is febrile and dehydrated. An intravenous infusion is established and Amy is to receive 3 L of fluid/m^2 of body surface area/day.

1 What is Amy's body surface area in m^2?

2 How much actual fluid/day should Amy receive from this order?

3 How many ml/hour should Amy receive from this infusion, and which method of delivery (a volumetric pump or a micro-dropper) would be more appropriate for its delivery?

Amy is given a statim dose of intravenous metoclopramide hydrochloride (Maxolon) for her vomiting. She is to have 100 mcg/kg of body weight.

4 What does the word 'statim' mean?

5 How many mg of Maxolon should Amy receive per dose?

6 If stock available is 5 mg/ml, what volume of this medication should be drawn up?

Amy is crying. She tells you that her 'tummy pains are really bad'. She is ordered intravenous pethidine, 2 mg/kg, to be given immediately, over a 3-minute period.

7 How much pethidine should she be given?

8 **a** From available stock of 100 mg/2 ml, what volume should be drawn up?
   b What type of syringe would be used to give this medication?

9 To try to reduce her fever, paracetamol elixir, 12 ml, 4-hourly PRN is ordered. How many mg of paracetamol will Amy receive for each dose if the concentration of the mixture is 24 mg/ml?

10 If the recommended dose of paracetamol is 15 mg/kg, 4-hourly, is the ordered dose within safe limits for Amy?

Next day when you return to duty, you learn at handover that Amy, who has just returned from an overseas holiday, has Typhoid Fever. She is ordered intravenous chloramphenicol (Chloromycetin) 25 mg/kg/day, to be administered every six hours

11 What is the daily dose of this medication for Amy?

12 How many mg should she receive for a single dose?

Chloromycetin is available as 1.2 g of powder in a vial. Instructions accompanying this medication indicate that 1.2 g of powder will displace one ml of fluid when reconstituted.

13 How much sterile water is required to make a concentration of 100 mg/ml?

14 What volume of medication should be drawn up for her first dose?

15 To prevent irritation of the vein, this medication is to be further diluted to a minimum concentration of 5%. How much fluid will be needed to achieve a 5% concentration if 10% is 100 mg/10 ml of solution?

16 A 50 ml bag of 0.9% sodium chloride is to be used to deliver the Chloromycetin and the registered nurse adds the prepared dose to this bag. Calculate how fast this medicated solution should drip at in order to complete in 30 minutes, if this line has a drop factor of 20 drops/ml.

When next you care for Amy, her condition has improved considerably. She is now tolerating fluids but the diarrhoea persists.

17 She is to have diphenoxylate (Lomotil) 8 mg/day in four equally divided doses for the diarrhoea. Stock available is 2 mg tablets. Calculate the number of tablets required for her 10.00 dose.

18 Oral Chloromycetin has now been ordered. She is to have chloromycetin palmitate which is available as 125 mg/5 ml of mixture. What volume should you pour for her midday dose if the dose, in mg, remains the same?

19 The intravenous infusion continues but the volumetric pump has been discontinued. Amy's infusion is dripping at the rate of 45 drops/minute via a micro-dropper. What volume of fluid is she receiving every hour from this infusion?

20 Amy is to have a minimum of 100 ml/hour today. Taking into account her infusion, how much oral fluid should you try to persuade Amy to drink every hour?

EXERCISE SIX

You are caring for six-month-old Nicky who has just returned to the ward following heart surgery two days ago. He weighs 5.6 kg.

1 An intravenous line is delivering 0.5 ml of 0.9% sodium chloride per minute via a volumetric pump. What volume of intravenous fluid is Nicky receiving each hour?

2 How long would you expect this 0.5 L bag to last?

A syringe pump is delivering morphine via a secondary line, to reduce his discomfort. The syringe contains 10 mg of morphine in 50 ml of fluid and is to last 40 hours.

3 What is the concentration, in mcg/ml, of this medicated solution?

4 How much morphine is Nicky receiving every hour?

5 An infant of Nicky's size can have up to 0.05 mg/kg/hour. Is the dose that he is receiving within these limits?

6 He is receiving intravenous digoxin (Lanoxin), 10 mcg/kg/day, which is given BD. If stock in the ward is 50 mcg/2 ml, how much medication should be drawn up for his morning dose?

On day three Nicky is commenced on nasogastric tube feeds of 80 ml of expressed breast milk. He is to have five feeds today at 06.00, 10.00, 14.00, 18.00 and 22.00. The drop factor for the tube feed giving set is 14 drops/ml and the feed should take one hour.

7 How fast, in drops/minute, should each feed drip?

8   An infant of Nicky's weight is permitted 100 ml of fluid per day per kg of body weight. Taking into account the breast milk he is receiving, how much fluid per hour should his intravenous infusion deliver to complement his milk and maintain a fluid intake within acceptable limits?

On day four his morphine infusion completes. He is now to have paracetamol elixir, 4 ml every 6 hours, if he is restless. This is to be introduced into his nasogastric tube at a 1 to 1 ratio using cooled boiled water as the solvent.

9   What volume of fluid, in relation to each administration of this medication, should be charted on his fluid balance chart?

10   If the paracetamol stock is 24 mg/ml, how many mg/dose is he receiving from this order?

11   What dosage, in mg, does he have each day if this medication is given every six hours, and is this dose within normal limits if he is permitted 15 mg/kg, every four hours?

It is day five and Nicky has just been breast fed by his mother. Because he is to continue with a strict fluid balance chart for the present, you are required to weigh him prior to and after his feed. His first weight was 5.62 kg and on completion of his feed, he weighed 5704 grams.

12   Bearing in mind that 1 ml is considered equal to 1 gram, what volume of breast milk did he receive for this feed?

13   Nicky is crying. You check his nappy and note that it is wet, so you change him and weigh the wet nappy. You are aware that the disposable nappy weighs 22 grams when dry, so what volume of urine should you chart on the output column of his fluid balance chart (FBC) if the wet nappy weighs 65 grams?

14   On day six, Nicky continues to be breast fed. If his feeds contain 105 ml, 122 ml, 95 ml, 110 ml and 125 ml, does he still need the intravenous line to meet his daily needs for fluid?

15   A premature infant weighing 800 grams is ordered intravenous gentamicin 5 mg/kg of body weight/day to be given in two equally divided doses. This medication is available with a concentration of 10 mg/ml. Calculate the volume to be drawn up and added to the intravenous infusion.

16   A child with a BSA of 0.6 m² is ordered 5 mg of a drug. If the recommended dose is 0.01 g/m², is this dose within normal limits?

17   An infant with epilepsy is ordered 50 mg of Dilantin per day, to be given 6/24. This child weighs 8.5 kg and the recommended dose of this medication is 5 mg/kg/day. Is this dose within normal limits?

18   An infant weighing 3.2 kg is ordered 30 mcg of Lanoxin, to be given BD. The recommended dose of Lanoxin for this child is 10 mcg/kg/day. Is this dose within normal limits?

19   You are caring for a very sick infant who weighs 9.6 kg. This infant, who is not currently taking any oral food or fluids, has an intravenous infusion in place, which is delivering 40 ml/hour via a volumetric pump. You are aware that children of less than 10 kg should have a fluid intake of 100 ml/kg/day. Is his current fluid intake appropriate?

20   A young child weighing 12 kg has an intravenous infusion delivering 20 ml/hour via a volumetric pump. This child is tolerating approximately 100 ml of milk every four hours. If he is permitted 1 L + 50 ml for every kg above 10 kg/day, is his fluid intake suitable for his requirements?

EXERCISE SEVEN

You are to assist with the care of two children, Juanita and Sally, under the guidance of a registered nurse. Five-year-old Juanita has an infected throat and Bronchitis. Her mother tells you that she is 3 feet 6 inches tall and her weight is 2 stone 9 ½ pounds.

1   Remembering that there are 14 pounds in each stone and that each kilogram equals 2.2 pounds, calculate her weight in kilograms.

2   Remembering that there are 12 inches in each foot and that each inch measures 2.54 cm, calculate her height in cm.

3   **a**   Juanita is to have Alclox (an antibiotic) to help fight her infection. She is to have 40 mg/kg/day, to be given 8-hourly. Calculate the total daily dose of this medication.

   b If stock available is a 100 ml bottle with a concentration of 125 mg/5 ml, what volume should be poured for a single dose?

4   Juanita is dehydrated and you have been asked to ensure that she has a copious fluid intake, a minimum of 1.6 L today, over a 12-hour period. How much fluid should you offer her every half hour?

5 **a** She is also febrile and has been ordered paracetamol elixir 15 mg/kg/dose to help to reduce her fever. How many mg/dose of this medication should she receive?

    b If stock of the above medication is available as a mixture with a concentration of 24 mg/ml, what volume should be poured?

    c This mixture that has just been poured is to be added to fruit juice, at a 1 in 5 ratio. Having done this, what volume of fluid should you offer her?

Juanita is refusing to drink the fluids that you offer her, despite the fact that you have tried to accommodate her tastes and wishes. After consultation with her medical officer, an intravenous line is established at 09.30. Juanita is to have 1.5 L of 0.9% sodium chloride over the next 24 hours.

6 **a** How many ml/hour should Juanita receive from this order?

    b If the drop factor for the giving set is 60 drops/ml, to what speed in drops/minute should the infusion be set?

7 **a** Juanita asks for an orange drink with water as the pure juice burns her throat, what volume of solute (orange juice) is required for a 150 ml glass of fluid at a 4:1 ratio?

    b How much ice water (solvent) should you add?

8 **a** Juanita is to have a 1 in 2 Cepacol gargle. If 15 ml of Cepacol is to be used, how much water is required for this task?

    b What instructions, with regard to the gargle, should be given to Juanita?

9   It is 13.00 and you have been asked to check Juanita's 1 L bag of intravenous infusion. You note that the fluid is dripping at 52 drops per minute and 880 ml remain in the bag. Is this infusion running to schedule?

The other child you are assisting with is seven-year-old Sally who is recovering from burns to 25% of her body surface area. Sally weighs 20 kg, is 115 cm tall and has a BSA of 0.8 m². Sally is being fed by a nasogastric tube as she is reluctant to eat and nutrients are essential for her burns to heal.

10 What is the actual surface area in m ² of Sally's burns?

11 Sally's normal caloric requirements are 1700 per day. If each calorie is equal to approximately 4 kilojoules, calculate her intake in kilojoules.

12 Sally is to have a 40% increase in her kilojoule intake to meet the metabolic demands incurred by the healing process of the burns. How many kilojoules (kj) should she have each day?

13 The commercially prepared product, Osmolite, has been ordered for Sally. Each 237 ml bottle has 1048 kj. Approximately how many bottles of this product are required each day to meet Sally's kilojoule requirements?

14 How many ml of fluid would the above feeds supply Sally with each day?

Because protein is essential for healing to take place, Sally's intake of this nutrient is to increase 200%. Each 237 ml bottle of Osmolite contains 8.8 grams of protein and Sally's usual requirements of protein are 1 gram/kilogram of body weight/day.

15 Are her protein requirements being met?

16 You have been asked to infuse a bottle of Sally's Osmolite over a 50-minute period. Bearing in mind that the drop factor for an Osmolite giving set is 14 drops/ml, to what speed should you adjust the rate of flow?

17 Following each feed, the nasogastric tube is flushed with 50 ml of water to remove food particles which could result in infection. Remembering the number of feeds that she is having each day (Q 13), how much fluid would be charted on her intake chart each day?

When you return to duty next morning, Sally has a continuous feed installed. Each 946 ml flask is to complete in nine hours and Sally has been ordered two flasks for today and a volumetric pump will control the rate of flow.

18 How many ml/hour should she receive from this order?

Sally is receiving an antibiotic to aid in the prevention and reduction of infection. She is to have Ceclor, 1 gram/m^2 of this medication per day, to be given 6-hourly.

19 **a** What is her daily dose of this medication?
  b How many mg constitute a single dose of this medication?

20 If the available stock of Ceclor is a 250 ml bottle with a concentration of 250 mg per 5 ml, what volume should be poured for her 10.00 dose?

EXERCISE EIGHT

Ten-year-old Lee has just been admitted to the ward with Pulmonary Tuberculosis. He is being nursed in a side room but is not considered to be infectious. He weighs 25 kg. He is to have a combination of drugs that are anti-tuberculotic, such as Isoniazid, Rifadin and Myambutol.

1 Lee is to have 6 mg/kg/day of Isoniazid. Stock available is 100 mg scored tablets and this medication to be given TDS. Calculate a single dose of medication.

2 He is also ordered Rifadin 10 mg/kg/day to be given each morning, half an hour before breakfast. Stock available is Rifadin syrup 100 mg/5 ml. How much mixture should be poured?

3 He is to have Myambutol daily. The initial dose is 24 mg/kg. Stock available is 100 mg and 400 mg tablets. Calculate this dose which is also to be given half an hour before breakfast, and indicate the tablet strength he should be given.

4 Myambutol is to continue daily but the rate is reduced to 8 mg/kg/day. With reference to the stock available (above), calculate his daily dose and state which tablets, and how many, he should be given.

5 A side effect of Isoniazid is a pyridoxine hydrochloride (Vitamin B_6) deficiency and so 37.5 mg of this drug (Vitamin B_6) is to be given daily. From available stock of 25 mg tablets, calculate the number of tablets he should be given each day.

6 He is also ordered Vitamin C, 0.75 g daily, to be given in three equally divided doses. Stock available is 500 mg flavoured (scored) tablets. Calculate the number of tablets he should be given for a single dose of Vitamin C.

Lee is considered to be thin for his age. However, as his appetite is good, his kilojoule intake is increased by 25%.

7 How many kilojoules should he have each day if his usual intake of 8800 kilojoules is increased by 25%?

8 10% of Lee's diet is to be devoted to protein. If each gram of protein is equivalent to 16 kilojoules, how many grams should be allocated to this nutrient each day?

9 30% of his diet is to be allocated to fat, preferably of vegetable origin. If each gram of fat is equal to 37 kilojoules, what is his daily fat intake in grams?

10 If complex carbohydrates will absorb 50% of his diet, how many kilojoules does he have left for sweets or simple carbohydrates?

Eight-year-old Lucy has been admitted to hospital with exacerbation of her Cystic Fibrosis condition. Lucy weighs 20 kg.

11 Lucy is to have 975 mg of Viokase per day, to be given TDS to aid in the digestion of her food. If stock available is 325 mg tablets, how many tablets should she be given/dose?

12 To reduce the gastric acidity of her stomach, Lucy is ordered cimetadine, 30 mg/kg of body weight/day, to be given TDS with the Viokase tablets. Stock on hand is 0.2 g tablets. What should she be given for her midday dose?

13 Salt depletion, due to excessive sweating, is also a problem for Lucy. She is encouraged to have 17.5 grams per week. How much salt should she have each day?

Because people with Cystic Fibrosis have impaired intestinal absorption, their dietary intake needs to be increased. Normally Lucy should consume approximately 7000 kilojoules each day but she is to have a 50% increase in her intake.

14 What would be her kilojoule intake now?

15 Lucy is to have 2 grams of protein/kg of body weight/day. If each gram of protein has approximately 16 kilojoules, how many kilojoules will be allocated to protein each day?

16 Children with Cystic Fibrosis often have trouble digesting fats, so Lucy's fat intake is reduced to 5% of her daily kilojoule intake. If each gram of fat has 37 kilojoules, how many grams of fat should she be allocated each day?

17 Lucy has a mild chest infection. She is to have the antibiotic, amoxycillin, 40 mg/kg of body weight/day, to be given 6-hourly. Stock available is 125 mg/5 ml Amoxil syrup. What volume should be poured for a single dose?

18 Lucy requires a bronchodilator to maintain an adequate airway. She is to have Bricanyl elixir 75 mcg/kg of body weight/dose. Stock in the ward is 0.3 mg/ml. Calculate the volume of a single dose of this medication.

19 If her breathing is very restricted, she may also use Bricanyl in a nebuliser. For this she may have 0.02 ml/kg of body weight/dose. What is the volume of this dose?

20 If Lucy uses the nebuliser, she is required to mix the above dose of Bricanyl with normal saline at a 1 in 5 ratio. How much fluid, in total, should be put into the nebuliser?

EXERCISE NINE

As part of your paediatric experience, you elect to spend a day in the Burns Unit. You are working with a registered nurse and caring for five-year-old Jenna who was admitted to the unit with burns to more than 20% of her body surface area following an incident where her nightgown caught fire when she was playing too near a heater. Jenna's mother tells you that Jenna is 115 cm in height and she weighs 20 kg.

On her admission to hospital at 08.00, an intravenous infusion is established, oxygen is commenced, and an indwelling urinary catheter is inserted. Assessment of Jenna's burns indicate that she has second degree burns to the front of both legs, the top of her right foot, her pubic area, abdomen and chest.

1   Using the nomogram provided in the appendix, calculate Jenna's body surface area in m².

2   With reference to the 'burns chart' for children (also in the appendix), calculate the percentage of body surface area burnt.

3   What is the actual surface area, in m², of her body that is burnt?

Her immediate fluid order for the first 24 hours is 4 ml of fluid × her weight in kg × the percentage of surface area burnt. She is to have half of this fluid in the first eight hours following her burns, which occurred at 07.30.

4   How much fluid will she have in the first 24 hours?

5   a   Remembering to take into account the time that the burns occurred, how much fluid should she have in the first eight hours following her injury?
    b   How many ml/hour should the volumetric pump deliver?

6   Jenna is ordered intravenous morphine for her pain. She is to have a statim dose of 0.15 mg/kg of body weight. Calculate the dose she should be given.

7   Available stock is 10 mg/ml, what volume should be drawn up?

Intravenous amoxycillin is ordered to minimise infection. Jenna is to have 40 mg/kg/day, to be given in four equally divided doses, via her infusion. The medication is available as 1 gram of powder in a 10 ml vial for reconstitution.

8   Calculate her daily dose of amoxycillin.

9   If the 1 g of powder occupies space equivalent to 0.7 ml, how much sterile water is required to reconstitute this medication to a concentration of 100 mg/ml?

10 What volume of amoxycillin is required for her first dose?

11 The above medication is to be added to a 50 ml bag of 0.9% sodium chloride connected to the main infusion as a 'secondary' line and infused over a 20-minute period. How fast should it drip if the drop factor for this line is 20 drops/ml?

Jenna calls you to tell you she is 'going to be sick'. She has an order for 3 mg of metoclopromide hydrochloride (Maxolon) syrup. Ward stock is a 100 ml bottle with a concentration of 1 mg/ml.

12 How much syrup should you pour if Jenna is to have a 3 mg dose?

A morphine infusion via a syringe driver is to be set up. You assist the registered nurses with this task. 24 mg of morphine is to be mixed with 0.9% sodium chloride to create a total volume of 48 ml which is to last for 24 hours.

13 If stock available is 10 mg/ml, what volume of morphine is required for this task?

14 How many ml of sterile 0.9% sodium chloride is needed to complete this task?

15 What is the concentration, in mg/ml, of this medicated solution?

16 How many ml per hour should be set on the syringe driver to deliver the prescribed dose?

At 12.30 you note that Jenna's urinary output has dropped to 20 ml over the last hour and you report this finding to the registered nurse.

17 If the expected urinary output for a child with burns is 2 ml/kg/hour for a child weighing less than 30 kg, is this drop in urinary output a concern to you?

Jenna is seen by the medical officer who orders the 0.9% sodium chloride to be replaced by 1 L of Ringer's Lactate solution.

18 **a** How much fluid should be charted on the intake column of the fluid balance chart for the four and a half hours the 0.9% sodium chloride was infusing?
  b You note that 286 ml remain in the flask. Is this the expected amount?

As Jenna's condition stabilises, a decision is made to 'tidy up' her burn wounds. Prior to the procedure, she is to have a bolus dose of 4 mg of morphine to be given over a 4-minute period.

19 **a** How many mg/minute has she been ordered for this procedure?

    b Remembering the concentration of this solution, how many ml of medicated solution will deliver the mg/minute that is required?

    c To what rate of flow will the syringe driver need to be altered to deliver the prescribed dose in the ordered time?

20 After her burns have been dressed, Jenna begins to vomit. An intravenous dose of Maxolon is now ordered. She is to have 2.5 mg. What volume of this medication is required if the stock available is 10 mg/2 ml?

EXERCISE TEN

Malcolm has been admitted to hospital with Asthma and Pneumonia. He has dyspnoea, a productive cough and is slightly cyanosed. He is 13 years old, weighs 55 kg and is 178 cm tall. He is commenced on oxygen and an intravenous line is established. You are caring for him today.

1 What is Malcolm's body surface area in m²?

2 **a** Malcolm is to have his first litre of 0.9% Sodium Chloride over a 6-hour period. How many ml/hour should he receive, and if the drop factor for the giving set is 20 drops/ml, how many drops per minute should be delivered?

    b If the infusion commenced at 07.40, at what time would you expect it to complete?

He is to have the antibiotic, flucloxacillin, to help combat his chest infection. A dose of 750 mg is to be given 6-hourly. This medication is available as 1 gram of powder in a 10 ml vial and the accompanying instructions tell you to add 3 ml of water to achieve a concentration of 250 mg/ml. The registered nurse is supervising you while you prepare the medication.

3 a What volume of solution will be in the vial when you add the sterile water?

  b How much solution should you draw up for his ordered dose?

This medicated solution is to be administered slowly via infusion and the registered nurse adds it to the 47 ml remaining in the burette.

4 a What is the concentration, in mg/ml, of the solution in the burette?

  b What rate of flow will deliver this medicated solution over a 30-minute period?

5 Malcolm is to have aminophylline (Cardophyllin) 200 mg, 6-hourly, to encourage bronchodilation. From available stock of 100 mg tablets, calculate the number of tablets he should be given per dose.

6 A Ventolin inhalation via a nebulizer has been ordered. He is to have 5 mg at a 1 in 2 ratio. If ward stock is 5 mg/ml, how much normal saline will need to be added?

7 It is 12.15 and you have been asked to go to lunch. However, you are keen to put up the new bag of fluid. You note that 100 ml remain in the bag and it is dripping at 58 drops per minute. Have you time for a 30-minute lunch break before this bag completes?

8 At 13.50 his bag 0.9% sodium chloride completes. 1 L of 5% dextrose is commenced and is to infuse at the rate of 2 ml/minute. How many drops per minute will deliver 2 ml/minute?

9 How many ml per hour is Malcolm receiving from this infusion, and when should you expect this bag to complete?

10 Following his evening meal, he complains of nausea. He is permitted 0.1 mg/kg/dose of oral prochlorperazine maleate (Stemetil). If stock available is 5 mg tablets, how many should he be given?

11 Malcolm requests 'something to help him to sleep'. He is ordered promethazine hydrochloride (Phenergan elixir) 12.5 mg. Stock available is 1 mg/ml. What volume of this medication should be poured for Malcolm?

You are also caring for Phillip, a 14-year-old boy who was admitted to the ward three weeks ago following a motor vehicle accident. His wounds include a compound fracture of the right tibia and fibula. Following surgery, to stabilise the fractures, he develops a methicillin-resistant staphlococcus aureus infection. You are to work out his medications for 10.00.

12 Amoxycillin, 3 g per day, is to be given 8-hourly. From available stock of 500 mg, how many capsules should you give him for his first dose?

13 Another antibiotic that he is to receive is ciprofloxacin (Ciproxin) 500 mg BD. From available stock of 0.25 g tablets, how many tablets should he have per dose?

14 Vitamin C is to be given to aid in stimulating his immune system and in the production of collagen formation for wound healing. He is to have 2 g per day, to be given QID. From ward stock of 250 mg tablets, how many tablets should be receive each dose?

His wound is debrided every morning at about 11.00. Prior to the commencement of this procedure he is permitted 30 mg of codeine PRN. You check first and ask if he requires this medication today and he assures you that he does.

15 From stock in hand of 30 mg tablets, how many tablets should you give him at 10.30 to prepare him for this painful procedure?

When you give him the codeine he informs you that although these tablets offer good pain relief, they are also very constipating. He asks if you will find out what he can have to alleviate this unpleasant side effect. You follow through with his request and phyllium (Metamucil) is ordered.

16 He asks you to explain how this medication will help to reduce his constipation. How should you respond?

17 If he is to begin with 28 g of this medication each day, to be given BD, and one rounded teaspoon equals 7 g, what should he be given each dose?

18 How should this medication be given so that he receives maximum effect from it?

When you visit him on your return from lunch, he asks for something for his headache. He tells you that the strain of having his wound attended to always leaves him tense. You are mindful of the fact that it is only three hours since he had the codeine. You check his medication sheet and note that paracetamol has been ordered PRN for pain.

19 Would you consider giving him the paracetamol?

20 If so, he is permitted 1 g, 4-hourly PRN and stock in the ward is 500 mg tablets. How many tablets should you give him?

 # ANSWERS

EXERCISE ONE

1　**a**　0.64 m² 　**b**　0.24 m² 　　**c**　1.28 m²

2　**a**　0.66 m² 　**b**　1.98 m² 　　**c**　0.44 m²

3　**a**　1.17 m² 　**b**　0.74 m² 　　**c**　0.1 m²

4　**a**　0.27 m² 　**b**　27 mg/day 　**c**　6.75 mg/dose 　**d**　1.35 ml/dose

5　**a**　1.0 m² 　**b**　200 mg/day 　**c**　5 ml

6　**a**　380 mg 　**b**　9.5 ml/dose

7　0.48 ml

8　**a**　480 mg 　**b**　6.4 ml

9　20 ml/dose

10　240 mg/dose

11　It is less than recommended. Connie could have up to 360 mg per dose.

12　90 ml

13　10 ml/dose

14　**a**　10 ml 　　**b**　This medication should be used with precaution if a penicillin allergy is present.

15 16 hours 40 minutes

16 **a** 960 mg/day   **b** 240 mg/dose   **c** 10 ml   **d** 2.4 ml

17 **a** 200 potential drops   **b** 12.5 days

18 **a** Yes   **b** 50 drops/min

19 160 ml of orange juice + 40 ml of water

20 9.6 ml/dose

EXERCISE TWO

1 $1\frac{1}{2}$ tablets

2 20 ml

3 125 ml/hour and 42 drops/minute

4 At 16.30. Yes, it is on schedule.

5 Yes (1.5 × 40 = 60 mg/dose × 6 doses)

6 4 ml

7 2 mg/ml

8 4 ml/hour

9 9.3 ml

10 5 ml

11 **a** 10 mg/ml   **b** 50 drops/minute

12 0.6 ml

13 **a** 2.5 mg/minute   **b** 1.25 ml/minute

14 75 ml/hour

15 100 ml/hour and 33 drops/minute

16 105 ml/hour and 28 drops/minute

17 150 ml

18 50 ml of cordial

19 2 capsules

20 $1\frac{1}{2}$ tablets

EXERCISE THREE

1 50 ml/hour and 50 drops/minute

2 15 mg/dose

3 0.3 ml

4 Check with 'MIMS' for dosage for a child of Stella's weight and age.

5 24 mg/ml should deliver a dose of 240 mg

6 Yes, this dose is 240 mg, and she is permitted up to 300 mg/dose.

7 500 mg

8 125 mg/dose

9 5 ml/dose

10 4 times per day

11 1/2 tablet

12 13 hours 20 minutes

13 25 drops/minute

14 800 mg/day

15 200 mg/dose

16 4.6 ml

17 2 ml/dose

18 1 suppository/dose

19 Yes. The concentration is now 200 mg in 50 ml or 4 mg/ml.

20 33 drops/minute

EXERCISE FOUR

1 0.58 m²

2 1450 ml or 1.45 L per day

3 60.4 ml/hr

4 900 mg/day

5 150 mg/dose

6 250 mg

7 2.3 ml of fluid

8 1.5 ml/dose

9 0.36 ml

10 0.72 ml

11 1.08 ml

12 360 mg/dose

13 90 mg/dose

14 16.87 ml or 17 ml

15 150 ml

16 240 mg/dose and 480 mg/dose

17 24 mg/ml (15 × 18 = 270)

18 100 ml/hour

19 It would be difficult to achieve an accurate intake using a micro-dropper at 100 drops/minute.

20 **a** 500 mg/dose   **b** 5 ml/dose

EXERCISE FIVE

1 0.8 m²

2 2400 ml or 2.4 L

3 100 ml/hour, using a volumetric pump because of the large volume/hour for this child.

4 Once only, give immediately

5 2.4 mg/dose

6 0.48 ml using an insulin syringe

7 48 mg

8 **a** 0.96 ml   **b** an insulin syringe

9 288 mg/dose

10 Yes (15 mg × 24 kg = 360 mg)

11 600 mg/day

12 150 mg/dose

13 11 ml of water

14 1.5 ml/dose

15 10% = 100 mg/10ml, 5% = 50 mg/10 ml. Dose is 150 mg in 30 ml.

16 34 drops/minute

17 1 tablet

18 6 ml

19 45 ml/hour

20 55 ml/hour

EXERCISE SIX

1 30 ml/hour

2 16 hours 40 minutes

3 200 mcg/ml

4 250 mcg/hour

5 Yes, he could have up to 280 mcg.

6 1.12 ml

7 19 drops/minute

8 6.66 ml/hour

9 8 ml/dose

10 96 mg

11 384 mg. Yes, he is permitted up to 504 mg/day.

12 84 ml this feed

13 43 ml of urine

14 He has had 557 ml, enough fluid for the day.

15 0.2 ml

16 Yes, $0.6 \times 10 = 6$ mg permitted

17 No, his dose is higher than normal since the dose for his weight is 42.5 mg/day.

18 Yes, $3.2 \times 10 = 32$ mcg/day

19 His intake is appropriate.

20 Yes. His intake is 1080 ml and he is permitted 1100 ml/day.

EXERCISE SEVEN

1 17 kg

2 106.68 cm

3 a 680 mg   b 9 ml

4 67 ml

5 a 255 mg   b 10.6 ml   c Approximately 53 ml

6 a 62.5 ml/hour   b 62 to 63 drops/minute

7 a 120 ml   b 30 ml

8 a 15 ml   b Be careful not to swallow the mixture—spit it out.

9 No, it is too slow—780 ml should be in the bag.

10 0.2 m²

11 6800 kilojoules

12 9520 kilojoules

13 9 bottles

14 2133 ml

15 Yes, more than required, she is receiving 79.2 grams.

16 66 drops/minute

17 2583 ml/day

18 105 ml/hour

19 **a** 800 mg   **b** 200 mg

20 4 ml/dose

EXERCISE EIGHT

1 50 mg/dose or ½ tablet

2 12.5 ml/dose

3 $1\frac{1}{2}$ × 400 mg tablets = 600 mg

4 Give 1/2 of a 400 mg tablet or 2 × 100 mg tablets

5 $1\frac{1}{2}$ tablets

6 1/2 tablet/dose

7 11 000 kilojoules

8 68.75 grams of protein

9 89 grams

10 1100 kilojoules for sweets

11 1 tablet/dose

12 1 tablet

13 2.5 grams/day

14 10 500 kilojoules/day

15 640 kilojoules/day

16 14 grams of fat

17 8 ml

18 5 ml/dose

19 0.4 ml

20 2 ml

EXERCISE NINE

1 0.8 m^2

2 29.75% of BSA

3 0.238 m^2

4 2380 ml/24 hours

5 a 1190 ml   **b** 158.66 ml/hour (note: burns occurred at 07.30 not 08.00)

6 3 mg

7 0.3 ml

8 800 mg

9 9.3 ml

10 2 ml

11 52 drops/minute

12 3 ml/dose

13 2.4 ml

14 45.6 ml

15 0.5 mg/ml

16 2 ml/hour

17 Yes, it is only half of the expected output.

18 **a** 714 ml   **b** Yes

19 **a** 1 mg/minute   **b** 2 ml   **c** 120 ml/hour for 4 minutes

20 0.5 ml

EXERCISE TEN

1 1.67 m^2

2 **a** 167 ml/hour and 56 drops/minute **b** At 13.40

3 **a** 4 ml   **b** 3 ml

4 **a** 15 mg/ml   **b** 33 drops/minute

5 2 tablets

6 1 ml

7 Yes, it should last 34 minutes at this rate of flow

8 40 drops/minute

9 120 ml/hour, it should complete at 22.10

10 1 tablet

11 12.5 ml

12 2 capsules

13 2 tablets

14 2 tablets

15 1 tablet

16 Metamucil adds bulk to the faeces, which in turn stimulates peristalsis.

17 2 teaspoons/dose, twice a day

18 Have it with a 250 ml glass of fluid and follow it with a further 250 ml of fluid.

19 Yes

20 2 tablets

5

Calculating Complex Volumes

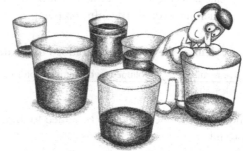

Objectives

After completing the given computations, it is expected that you should be able to:

1 enhance the speed at which you complete previously learnt calculations

2 calculate safe dosages of medications for all the clients in your care

3 manage complex intravenous infusions, including those requiring additives

EXERCISE ONE

CALCULATING COMPLEX VOLUMES IN ML/HOUR

Should you be working in a specialised area of nursing, you may be required to work out a complicated formula for medication administration.

 Example

Jimmy Richards is brought into the Emergency Department with multiple injuries following a motor vehicle accident. As part of his resuscitation regime, he is to have a Dopamine infusion of 4 mcg/kg/minute. Jimmy weighs 60 kg. The solution to be made up consists of 400 mg of dopamine hydrochloride and 250 ml of 5% dextrose. Stock available is a 10 ml ampoule with a concentration of 40 mg/ml.

1 Calculate the volume to be added to the dextrose.
2 Calculate the rate of flow (in ml/hour) required to deliver this order via a volumetric infusion pump.

1 Calculate the volume to be added to the dextrose

$$\frac{\text{Dose required}}{\text{Stock available}} \times \frac{\text{Volume in which it is dissolved}}{1} = \frac{400}{40} \times \frac{1}{1} = 10$$

The volume of medication to be added to the 250 ml of 5% dextrose is 10 ml.

2 Calculate the rate of flow required to deliver the order

$$\frac{\text{Dose required}}{\text{Dose in solution}} \times \frac{\text{Volume in which this dose is dissolved}}{1}$$

$$\frac{4 \text{ mcg} \times 60 \text{ kg} \times 60 \text{ mins}}{400\,000 \text{ mcg}} \times \frac{260 \text{ ml}}{1} \quad (250 \text{ ml} + 10 \text{ ml}) = 9.36$$

The volume of this medicated solution that should be administered to this client is 9.36 ml/hour.

Activity

Complete the following computations by indicating the **volume/hour** required to fulfil the given orders

1   Drug A is to be infused at the rate of 15 mcg/kg/minute for a 70 kg client. The prepared stock of 100 ml contains 400 mg of drug A.

2   Drug B is to be infused at the rate of 4 mg/minute. The prepared stock contains 1 g of drug B in a 100 ml solution.

3   Drug C is to infuse at the rate of 1 mg/kg/hour for a 60 kg person. The prepared stock contains 10 g of drug C in 500 ml of solution.

4   Your client is to have 10 mcg/minute of noradrenalin. The prepared stock contains 6 mg of noradrenalin in 100 ml of 5% dextrose. Calculate the rate of flow in ml/hour.

5   A 65 kg client has been ordered a sodium nitroprusside infusion of 3 mcg/kg/minute. The prepared stock that is available contains 50 mg of sodium nitroprusside in a 500 ml solution. Calculate the rate of flow in ml/hour.

6   A client receiving a Heparin infusion is to have 1250 units/hour. The prepared infusion contains 25 000 units of Heparin in 500 ml of 0.9% sodium chloride. Calculate the rate of flow, in ml/hour, for this order.

7   A client with severe burns is to receive 25 mg of pethidine per hour, via an infusion pump. This infusion contains 500 mg of pethidine in 100 ml of 5% dextrose. At what speed (in ml/hour) should the volumetric pump be set to deliver this order?

8   A client is to have 30 mg of Aminophylline per hour. Stock in use is 750 mg of Aminophylline in 1 L of 5% dextrose. Calculate the rate of flow, in ml/hour, for this order.

9   A client weighing 50 kg is to receive 2 units/kg/minute of Heparin. The prepared stock contains 18 000 units of Heparin in 100 ml of 0.9% sodium chloride. How many ml/hour should the volumetric pump deliver to fulfil this order?

Frequently, solutions are made up by mixing a powder with a fluid at a weight/volume (W/V) ratio. **It should be assumed, unless stated otherwise, that when the solution is formed, 1 gram of powder will displace 1 ml of fluid.** So, in a 10% solution of 100 ml, the weight of the powder should be 10 grams and the fluid contribution would be 90 ml.

For the following solutions, write the weight of the solute in grams and the volume of the solvent in ml.

10 **a** 100 ml with a 10% concentration
    b 100 ml with a 25% concentration
    c 100 ml with a 30% concentration
    d 100 ml with a 50% concentration

11 **a** 250 ml with a 20% concentration
    b 250 ml with a 10% concentration
    c 250 ml with a 40% concentration
    d 250 ml with a 30% concentration

You are caring for a client who weighs 60 kg. This person is to have 150 mg/kg of body weight of drug A over a 30-minute period. The medication is available as a 10% solution in a 100 ml bag, and is to be delivered via a volumetric pump in ml/hour.

12 What is the dose of this order in grams?

13 How many grams of drug A is there in this 100 ml bag?

14 What volume of this solution will you need to infuse?

15 To what speed, in ml/hour, will you need to set the pump to deliver the ordered dose in the prescribed time?

You have been asked to assist in the care of a client who has just returned to the ward from the Intensive Care Unit (ICU), where he was managed for multiple injuries following a motor vehicle accident. A pethidine infusion is to be established for pain control, and the dose requirement is 0.5 g in a 100 ml bag of 0.9% sodium chloride, to last 25 hours. Pethidine is available in 2 ml ampoules with a concentration of 100 mg/2 ml and the infusion is to be delivered by a volumetric infusion pump.

16 What volume of pethidine should be drawn up for this task?

17 If the total volume required is 100 ml, how much fluid will need to be removed from the bag before the medication is added?

18 **a** What is the concentration, in mg/ml, of this medicated solution?
   b To what speed, in ml/hour, should the volumetric pump be set?

Two hours later, this client rings his call bell and asks if the pain medication could be increased as his pain is severe. An order is given for him to receive a bolus dose of 12 mg of pethidine over a 4-minute period, and then he is to return to his usual dose rate.

19 **a** How many mg/minute should he receive from this new order?
   b What volume of medicated solution contains the ordered mg/minute?
   c To what speed, in ml/hour, should you adjust the infusion pump to deliver the bolus dose in the prescribed time?

20 Calculate the rate of flow, in ml/hour, for the following
   a 5000 units in 1 L, to be delivered at the rate of 500 units/hour
   b 1 000 000 units in 250 ml, to be delivered at the rate of 500 000 units/hour
   c 1 gram in 0.5 L, to be delivered at the rate of 200 mg/hour
   d 1.5 g in 1 L, to be delivered at the rate of 75 mg/hour
   e 750 mg in 250 ml, to be delivered at the rate of 150 mg/hour

EXERCISE TWO

You have just come on duty for a morning shift and you are to care for 18-year-old Van Tran who is a newly arrived migrant from an overseas refugee camp. She has been hospitalised following a diagnosis of Tuberculosis. Van is very thin and frail, her height is 155 cm and her weight is 40 kg.

To avoid the possibility of the Tuberculosis bacillus becoming resistant to the drug therapy, a combination of drugs is administered in the initial period of Van's treatment.

1 At 07.30 Van begins her daily medication regime. Rifampicin (Rifadin) is ordered, 0.45 g is to be given daily, half an hour before breakfast. Stock in hand is 150 and 300 mg capsules. What should she be given?

2 a In conjunction with Rifadin, Van is to have Isoniazid (INH) 5 mg/kg of body weight/day, to be given 6-hourly. Calculate the daily dose of this medication.

b From available stock of 100 mg scored tablets, calculate a single dose for her.

3 Pyrazinamide (Zinamide) 25 mg/kg/day is also to be given 6-hourly. Stock available is 0.5 scored tablets. Calculate her 10.00 dose.

4 Ethambutol (Myambutol) at 20 mg/kg is to be given daily in a single dose. Stock in the ward is 400 mg tablets. Calculate her 12.00 dose.

Because people receiving Isoniazid therapy excrete large amounts of Pyridoxine (Vitamin B_6), this nutrient must be replaced to prevent the possible development of neuritis. Van is to have 50 mg daily, to be given BD.

5 From available stock of scored 50 mg tablets, what should she be given?

6 Van is considered undernourished and she is to have a high carbohydrate, high vitamin and high protein diet. If the acceptable weight for someone of Van's weight is 50 kg, by what percentage is she considered underweight?

7 Van's diet is to include a minimum of 2250 calories per day. If each calorie is equal to approximately four kilojoules, how many kilojoules per day should she have?

8 Her diet is to include 1.5 grams of protein per kg of ideal body weight each day. What percentage of her diet will be protein if one gram of protein equals 16 kilojoules?

9 A maximum of 28% of Van's diet is to be fat, preferably from a vegetable source. Remembering that each gram of fat equals 37 kilojoules, approximately how many grams of fat will she have each day?

10 How many kilojoules remain for her carbohydrate intake?

11 60% of the carbohydrate should be of the complex variety type. How many grams will this be if one gram of carbohydrate equals 16 kilojoules?

12 How many kilojoules are left for simple sugars such as sweets?

Mr Psanka has been admitted to the ward with Acute Gastritis. His nursing notes state that he has a history of taking large doses of aspirin to relieve the pain of a previous back injury. He has epigastric pain, vomiting, diarrhoea and is dehydrated.

13 An intravenous line is established and 1 L of 0.9% sodium chloride is to infuse at the rate of 0.2 L per hour. How long would you expect this flask to last?

14 If the drop factor for the giving set is 20 drops/ml, what should be the rate of flow in drops/minute?

Mr Psanka says he feels nauseated and faint. You take his blood pressure and note that the systolic reading is 90 and the diastolic reading is 50. Before you have time to report this, he vomits a large amount of partially clotted blood. His pulse is rapid and weak, his skin cold and clammy. He is seen by a medical officer and blood is to be urgently cross-matched.

15 Meanwhile, 500 ml of Haemaccel is commenced and is to complete in two hours. How many drops per minute are required to deliver this rate of flow?

16 **a** 0.5 L of whole blood arrives and is commenced as soon as the Haemaccel completes. The initial rate of flow is 15 drops per minute. If this rate of flow is to continue for 15 minutes, how much blood will he receive in this time?
   b If there is no evidence of a transfusion reaction, the remainder of the blood is to infuse at the rate of 2 ml/minute. If the blood commenced at 11.30, when would you expect it to complete?
   c How many drops/minute are needed to deliver 2 ml/minute?

Ranitidine hydrochloride (Zantac) is to be given intravenously today. He is to have 0.2 g/day, to be given 6-hourly on completion of the transfusion.

17 **a** From available stock of 50 mg/2 ml, calculate the volume of a single dose of this medication.

  b This medication is to be added to 20 ml of normal saline in the burette and infused over a 10-minute period. How fast should it drip?

18 Next day when you return to duty Mr Psanka's condition has improved considerably. Oral Zantac has replaced the previous day's intravenous dose. He is to have 150 mg BD. From stock equivalent to 0.15 g, how many tablets should he be given?

19 On day three, Mr Psanka can have diluted apple juice. How much solvent is required to make 300 ml of a 4 in 5 solution of juice?

20 Mr Psanka is ready to go home. Pharmacy has sent up a 500 ml bottle Amphojel. If he is to have 10 ml of this medication five times per day, how long will this bottle last?

EXERCISE THREE

You are caring for seventeen-year-old Paul who has been admitted to the ward with severe Pneumonia. He tells you he has no fixed abode and admits to being an intravenous drug user. On admission he has chest pain and marked respiratory distress. He is flushed and dehydrated. Oxygen is commenced.

1 An intravenous line is established with 5% dextrose, 1 L is to infuse at the rate of 4 ml/minute for the first hour. If the drop factor is 20 drops/ml, how many drops/minute will need to infuse?

2 **a** Intravenous erythromycin (an antibiotic) is commenced. The ordered dose is 60 mg/kg/day. Paul tells you that he weighs 7 stone 12 pounds. If there are 14 pounds per stone and 2.2 pounds per kg, what is his weight in kg?
  b Calculate the daily dose of this medication.
  c How many mg/dose should he receive if the medication is to be given 6-hourly?

3 **a** The stock of erythromycin is 1 g of powder in a 10 ml vial. If the 1 g occupies the space of 1 ml, how much sterile water needs to be added to the vial to make a concentration of 100 mg/ml?

b What volume of medication should be drawn up for his first dose?

4 In order to reduce venous irritation, the medication is added to 100 ml of 0.9% sodium chloride via a secondary line with a drop factor of 20 drops/ml, and is to infuse over an hour. How many drops per minute will deliver this order?

5 Paul is ordered 70 mg of pethidine for his chest pain. From available stock of 100 mg/2 ml, calculate the volume you should give him.

6 **a** Paul's infusion rate has been reduced to 2 ml/minute. To what speed should you adjust the drops/minute?
   b Taking into account the rate of flow for the first hour, how long would you expect the remainder of this bag to last?

During your routine observations of this young man you record a temperature of 39.8°C. You are asked to give him 0.6 g of dispersible aspirin. When you take the medication to him and tell him what it is, he refuses to have it.

7 **a** Explain to Paul the reason why the aspirin has been ordered.
   b These tablets are to be given in a mixture of not less than 10 mg/ml. How much water should you dissolve these tablets in?

8 A cough expectorant has been ordered. Paul is to have Mist Potassium Iodide QID. Stock in the ward is a 200 ml bottle containing 25 mg/ml. Calculate his 14.00 dose if he is to have 1.2 g/day.

9 Because Paul is so dehydrated, you are to encourage oral fluids. He is to drink 1 L each day while his intravenous line is in place. How could the fluid be evenly distributed between the hours of 06.00 and 22.00?

10 Paul refuses the water in his jug. You make up some cordial for him. The instructions advise you to mix 200 ml of cordial to 800 ml of water. Write this mixture as a ratio___ in___.

11 Two hours after the pethidine was given, Paul becomes angry and aggressive. He demands another dose as 'this has done no

good at all'. Why might this medication have been less than effective?

12 Paul is seen by the medical officer who orders another 100 mg of pethidine. With reference to Q 5 for available stock, what volume of pethidine should you draw up?

13 On completion of the 5% dextrose, 1 L of 0.9% sodium chloride is commenced. Calculate the rate of flow in drops per minute if this flask is to last six hours.

During visiting hours Paul asks you to close the curtain so he can talk to his girlfriend in private. When she leaves, you check to see if Paul has settled. He does not respond. His pupils are pinpoint, his breathing is almost imperceptible, his skin is cold and clammy. You ring the buzzer for emergency assistance.

14 The registered nurse who answers your call asks you to draw up 0.8 mg of naloxone (a narcotic antagonist). Stock available on the emergency trolley is 400 mcg/ml. What volume should you draw up?

15 Paul responds to a second dose of naloxone, but a decision is made to add this drug to his 0.9% sodium chloride infusion, which has 500 ml remaining. A solution containing 2 mg is injected into the infusion. What is the concentration (in mcg/ml) of this medicated solution?

16 If Paul is to receive 400 mcg/hour, how many ml/hour will the volumetric pump need to deliver to fulfil this order?

Paul's condition has markedly improved when you return to duty in two days time. His intravenous erythromycin has been replaced by oral erythromycin, and the dose has been reduced to 1.5 g/day.

17 Stock in hand is 250 mg capsules. What should you give him at 10.00 if his medication is to be given 8-hourly?

18 Paul is experiencing difficulty expelling sputum. A Mucomyst inhalation is ordered to alter the viscosity of his sputum. He is to have 3 ml of Mucomyst at a 1 to 1 ratio with normal saline four times per day. What volume of fluid should you end up with in the nebuliser?

19 Paul's intravenous infusion can be removed and he can leave the hospital when the present bag completes. If 90 ml remain in the bag and it is dripping at 20 drops/minute, how much longer is Paul required to remain in hospital?

20 He is to continue the erythromycin for another seven days, at the rate of 1 gram/day. How many 250 mg capsules will pharmacy need to dispense for this order?

EXERCISE FOUR

Mrs Pamela Clark has been admitted to the ward for a total hip replacement following a fall where she fractured the neck of her left femur. She has a history of Deep Vein Thrombosis and Hypertension. She tells you that she has been on 'the pill' for years and she smokes 25 cigarettes each day. Her weight is 62 kg.

1 At 22.00, Mrs Clark requests night sedation. Nitrazepam 10 mg is ordered. Calculate the number of tablets to be given if available stock is 5 mg/tablet.

2 At 08.00 next morning an intravenous infusion of Compound Sodium Lactate (Hartman's solution) is commenced. The 1 L bag is to complete in six hours. If the drop factor is 20 drops/ml, calculate the rate of flow in drops per minute.

3 Her premedication is due. She is to have 100 mg of pethidine and 400 mcg of Atropine. From available stock of 100 mg/2 ml, how much pethidine should you draw up?

4 Atropine is available as 0.5 mg/ml. What volume do you require?

5 Mrs Clark returns to the ward at 12.30. The intravenous bag contains 250 ml of Hartman's solution. Is this infusion running to schedule?

Because Mrs Clark has a history of Deep Vein Thrombosis, has been taking the contraceptive pill and is a cigarette smoker, she is considered to be at great risk of developing another Deep Vein Thrombosis. She is to have continuous intravenous Heparin for 24 hours while she is immobile. 5000 units is added to the 1 L of 0.9% sodium chloride which is to commence at 14.00.

6 Calculate the rate of flow (via a volumetric pump) for this infusion if Mrs Clark is to receive 625 units per hour.

At 14.15, you assist the registered nurses to set up a morphine infusion via a syringe driver for Mrs Clark. She is to have 60 mg of morphine in a 60 ml solution which is to last for 24 hours.

7 a From available stock of 15 mg/ml, what volume of this solution will be morphine?
   b How much 0.9% sodium chloride is required to complete this task?
   c What is the concentration (mg/ml) of this medicated solution?
   d How many ml/hour will deliver the ordered dose in 24 hours?

Mrs Clark is nauseated. She is ordered metoclopramide (Maxolon) and may have up to 30 mg per day. This medication can be given intravenously, 4-hourly PRN. Stock on hand is 10 mg/2 ml.

8 What volume should be drawn up for her first dose?

9 If the recommended daily dose of Maxolon is 0.5 mg/kg, is Mrs Clark's dose within normal limits?

Flucloxacillin (Flopen) is ordered as a prophylactic measure against infection. Mrs Clark is to have 3 grams per day, to be given intravenously every six hours. This drug is available as 1 g of powder in a 10 ml vial and instructions accompanying the medication indicate that the powder will displace 1 ml of fluid when reconstituted.

10 a How much sterile water is required to make a concentration of 100 mg/ml when you take into account the 1 g of medication in the 10 ml vial?
   b How many mg/dose should Mrs Clark receive?
   c What volume should be drawn up for her 16.00 dose?
   d You are to add the ordered dose to 20 ml of infusion solution into the burette and deliver the antibiotic over a 15-minute period. How many drops/min are required for this task?

11 Verapamil hydrochloride (Isoptin) is prescribed to lower Mrs Clark's blood pressure. She is to have 240 mg per day, to be given BD. From available stock of 40, 80, 120 and 160 mg tablets, calculate what she should be given at 18.00.

When you return to duty next morning, you are again to care for Mrs Clark. The third 1 L bag of 0.9% sodium chloride with added Heparin is infusing at 125 ml/hr.

12 Is this the recommended rate of flow for this infusion?

13 Mrs Clark's nausea has subsided and bowel sounds are present. At 09.00, oral fluids are introduced. She may have 30 ml of iced water per hour for the next four hours. How much fluid will be charted in the oral intake column of her fluid balance chart if she drinks it all?

Following her morning sponge, Mrs Clark asks for a 'stronger pain killer'. She is ordered a bolus dose of 3 mg of morphine over a 3-minute period.

14 a How many mg/minute are required to deliver the bolus dose in the prescribed time?
   b What volume of fluid per minute will deliver your calculated dose?
   c To what speed, in ml/hr, will you need to adjust the infusion pump to accommodate the new order?

15 At 14.00 the Heparin infusion ceases and is replaced with a 5% dextrose solution. This flask is to last ten hours. Calculate the rate of flow in drops/minute.

16 Mrs Clark notes the dextrose infusion and asks you how much 'glucose' is in the 1 L bag. How many grams of dextrose is in this 5% solution?

17 How many kilojoules will this solution supply to Mrs Clark if 1 g of dextrose has four calories and each calorie has approximately 4 kilojoules?

18 Mrs Clark is up and mobilising with assistance. Her Heparin is reduced to 4000 units BD. If stock available is 5000 units/0.2 ml, what volume should be measured (using a 0.5 ml insulin syringe) for her 10.00 subcutaneous injection?

19 She asks for pain relief prior to her morning shower. She is ordered 45 mg of codeine. If stock in hand is 30 mg tablets, what should she be given?

20 Oral Flopen is to replace the intravenous medication. The dose has been reduced to 2 g/day, to be given 6-hourly. From available stock of 250 mg capsules, what should she be given for her 12.00 dose?

EXERCISE FIVE

Mrs Kitson is a 60-year-old woman weighing 55 kg who has been admitted to the ward for bowel surgery in two days time. On admission she is anxious and tells you that she is 'far too concerned about her illness to sleep tonight'. You are to care for Mrs Kitson under the guidance of the registered nurse.

1 Diazepam (Valium) 10 mg is ordered to allay anxiety. From available ward stock of 5 mg tablets, what should she be given?

Next morning when you return to duty, you are to follow through with the care of Mrs Kitson. She is commenced on oral antibiotics to reduce the microbial population in her bowel. She is to have 1 g of neomycin every hour for four hours. Stock available is 500 mg tablets.

2 How many tablets should she be given every hour?

3 a She is then to have 1 g every four hours for another four doses. How many neomycin tablets will she have in total?
   b How many grams of neomycin has she had?

At 14.00 she is commenced on a medication to cleanse her bowel. At this point in time, she is asked to consume only low or fibre-free foods (to reduce the faecal content in her bowel) and fluids until after her operation. An intravenous infusion is established to combat dehydration. The 1 L of 0.9% sodium chloride is to infuse at the rate of 200 ml per hour.

4 How long would you expect this bag of fluid to last and how many drops/minute will deliver this order if the drop factor for the giving set is 20 drops/ml?

5   On day three, just prior to her operation, Mrs Kitson is given a bowel washout. The amount of fluid introduced into her bowel is 4 L and the measured return on completion of the task is 3.6 L. What should be charted on her input and output chart (in mls)?

6   A premedication to enhance drowsiness is due, and 75 mg of pethidine is to be given. If stock on the ward is 50 mg/ml, what volume should be drawn up?

7   The medication ordered to reduce her respiratory secretions is Atropine 0.4 mg. If stock on hand is 500 mcg/ml, what volume is required?

Following the administration of her premedication at 09.00, you check her intravenous infusion. You note that there is 90 ml of 0.9% sodium chloride in the bag and it is dripping at 60 drops per minute.

8   Have you time to complete a lengthy dressing procedure (approximately 30 minutes) before the bag completes?

9   a   Mrs Kitson returns to the ward at 13.30 following resection of a malignant tumour in her transverse colon. Her present bag of 5% dextrose is infusing at the rate of 2 ml/minute. How long would you expect the remaining 180 ml to last?
    b   How many drops per minute will deliver 2 ml/minute?

An infusion is to be set up to help control her pain. You are observing two registered nurses preparing this medicated solution. 400 mg of pethidine is to be dissolved in a solution of 0.9% sodium chloride. A 100 ml bag is to be used for this purpose.

10   a   From available stock of 100 mg/2 ml, what volume of pethidine will need to be drawn for this procedure?
    b   What volume of fluid is in the bag when the medication is added?
    c   If this medicated solution is to last for 24 hours, to what speed, in ml/hour, will the volumetric pump need to be set?
    d   What is the concentration, in mg/ml, of this medicated solution?
    e   How much pethidine will Mrs Kitson receive every four hours?

f If the recommended maximum adult dose of intravenous pethidine is 50 mg every three hours, is the ordered dose of pethidine that she is receiving within acceptable limits?

Although Mrs Kitson has a nasogastric tube which is connected to low continuous gastric suction, she tells you that she is nauseated and feels as though she is going to vomit. Consultation with the medical officer caring for her, results in an order for intravenous metoclopramide (Maxolon) 7.5 mg, 6-hourly PRN.

11 From available stock of 10 mg/2 ml, what volume of medication should be drawn up for her first dose?

Mrs Kitson continues to state that she 'feels awful' and that her pain is severe. A decision is made to give her a bolus dose of intravenous pethidine over a 4-minute period. The registered nurse increases the rate of flow (via the volumetric pump) to 60 ml/hour for four minutes and then returns the rate of flow back to the original order.

12 a How many ml/minute will the bolus dose deliver?
  b How many mg of pethidine are in one ml of this medicated solution?
  c How many mg of pethidine will this bolus dose deliver?

As a prophylactic measure against infection, Mrs Kitson is to continue an antibiotic regime. She is to have intravenous gentamicin, 3 mg/kg/day, to be given in a single dose.

13 a From available stock of 80 mg/2 ml, what volume should be drawn up for this order?
  b This medication is to be administered at a concentration no greater than 2 mg/ml. How much fluid will need to be in the burette to achieve this concentration?
  c Calculate the rate of flow in drops/minute if this medication is to infuse over a 30-minute period.

At 15.00 her present bag of 5% dextrose completes. You check her fluid order sheet and note that she is to have 3 L of normal saline over the next 24 hours and 1 g of potassium chloride is to be added to each 1 L bag. Potassium chloride (KCl) is available as 0.75 g/10 ml.

14 a What volume of potassium chloride should be drawn up to be added to the 1 L of normal saline?

b What is the concentration, in mg/ml, of potassium chloride to sodium chloride for the first bag of this order?

c How many ml/hour are required? Calculate the drops/minute that will fulfil this order?

d What specific observations of Mrs Kitson will you need to make while KCl is being administered?

When you return to duty next morning, you note that blood has been ordered for Mrs Kitson. You visit her on completion of handover at 07.30 and she tells you that she still feels nauseated and has cramp-like pains in her abdomen. You note that the drainage from the nasogastric suction is free and the drainage bottle contains 300 ml, which has accumulated since 06.00 that morning. Her urinary catheter bag, also last emptied at 06.00, has 25 ml. Her intravenous infusion is dripping at 52 drops/minute.

15 a How many ml of urine per hour would you expect this client to produce?

b Is the intravenous infusion dripping at the prescribed rate?

c You take her blood pressure and note that it has dropped from 145/90 to 105/65. Would you consider this to be of concern in relation to the medications she is receiving?

d What actions should you take with regard to your findings?

Mrs Kitson is seen by the medical officer and following an evaluation of her serum electrolytes, the potassium chloride is discontinued. You are asked to remove the existing bag of saline and line and replace it with a new line primed with 50 ml 0.9% sodium chloride as her blood has arrived.

16 a Why have you been asked to infuse this 50 ml of 0.9% sodium chloride when a saline solution was already in progress?

b As you check the blood with the registered nurse, Mrs Kitson makes the comment that it is a small amount of blood. Explain to her the difference between whole blood and packed cells.

c The blood is commenced at 1 ml/minute. Why is this so?

d After fifteen minutes, the rate of flow is increased to 2.5 ml/minute. How many drops will deliver 2.5 ml/minute?

When the blood completes, you are asked to infuse a 100 ml bag of 0.9% sodium chloride over 30 minutes, and then commence 1 L of 5% dextrose which is to last ten hours.

17 a Why does the 0.9% sodium chloride need to precede the dextrose solution?

   b What is the rate, in drops/minute, for the 0.9% sodium chloride?

   c How fast should the dextrose drip?

When you return to duty on day three, post-surgery, Mrs Kitson is looking much better. She tells you that the suction has been discontinued and she can have some ice to suck.

18 a What assessment of Mrs Kitson would indicate that fluids could begin?

   b Ice chips, 30 ml per hour, are given from 08.00 until 12.00 with no ill effects. How much fluid will be charted on the fluid balance chart in her oral intake column, in relation to ice chips?

Her nasogastric tube is removed and clear fluids, as tolerated, may be given. She asks you to dilute her tin of pulp-free orange juice at a ratio of 3:2.

19 How much ice water is required to make up a 250 ml glass of orange juice?

20 The intravenous gentamicin has been reduced to 80 mg daily. From stock on hand of 40 mg/ml, what volume will be drawn up for her 10.00 dose?

EXERCISE SIX

At 06.30 Mr Don Adams was admitted to the ward with severe Gastro-enteritis. He was vomiting and had diarrhoea, his colour was flushed and he showed signs of dehydration. At 07.00 when you come on duty, you are assigned to care for him. On admission his weight is 60 kg.

1 Remembering that there are 14 pounds to one stone and that 2.2 pounds make one kg, convert his weight to stones and pounds.

2 Mr Adams tells you that he normally weighs 10 stone. Calculate his weight loss and express this as a fluid loss.

An intravenous infusion is established. He is to have 3 L over the next 21 hours. While the order for this fluid is clearly set out, the registered nurse asks you to 'problem solve' this intake, which is to be delivered via a volumetric pump. For example, in this order, the second bag of fluid is to run at half the speed of the first bag and the third bag is to infuse at half the speed of the second bag. All are to complete within 21 hours.

3   Calculate the ml/hour the first bag will deliver.

4   How many ml/hour will the second bag deliver?

5   Bag number three will deliver how many ml/hour?

Mr Adams is ordered metoclopramide hydrochloride (Maxolon) for his nausea and vomiting. He is to have 0.5 mg/kg of body weight/day, to be given intravenously every six hours PRN.

6   **a**   How much Maxolon is he permitted per day and how many mg/dose should he receive if the medication is to be given 6-hourly?
     b   If stock available is 10 mg/2 ml, what volume should you draw up for his first dose?

At 08.00, intravenous amoxycillin sodium (Amoxyl), the antibiotic ordered to combat his gastro-intestinal infection, is commenced. He is to have 1 gram every eight hours. Stock available is 1 g of powder in a 10 ml vial. Instructions accompanying this medication indicate that by adding 4.3 ml of sterile water you will achieve a concentration of 200 mg/ml.

7   **a**   After adding the water, what is the total volume of solution in the vial?
     b   What volume of solution per dose is required to fulfil the order?

8   This medication that you have just prepared is to be added to a 50 ml bag of 0.9% sodium chloride and delivered over a 20-minute period. Calculate the rate of flow, in drops/minute, for the infusion if the drop factor is 20 drops/ml.

During a routine check of Mr Adam's condition, you note that his pulse is irregular and his respirations are quite shallow, and he tells you that he feels very weak. Evaluation of his electrolyte status indicates a depletion of potassium stores (Hypokalaemia). Potassium chloride is ordered, to be added to 100 ml of 0.9% sodium chloride and commenced via the secondary line when his antibiotic completes.

9 You observe the registered nurse preparing the 100 ml bag of 0.9% sodium chloride which is to have 0.5 gram of potassium chloride added. From available stock of 750 mg/10 ml, what volume of potassium should she draw up?

10 The potassium chloride is to infuse at the rate of 1.5 mg per minute. How long would you expect this 100 ml bag to last, and how many drops/minute will deliver the ordered dose if the drop factor for the giving set is 60 drops/ml?

At 10.00 Mr Adams rings his bell to tell you that his abdominal pain, which is colicky in nature, is becoming unbearable. You note that his colour is pale and his skin is cool and clammy. He is ordered 12 mg of morphine statim.

11 a What does the word 'statim' mean?
   b From available stock of 15 mg/ml, how much morphine should you draw up?

Mr Adams settles after the morphine injection and when you next find him awake, he tells you that he feels much better. Diphenoxylate (Lomotil), 20 mg/day, is ordered, to be given 6-hourly. This medication is related to pethidine and acts by slowing intestinal motility.

12 Calculate a single dose of Lomotil, and from available stock of 2.5 mg tablets, what should he be given?

When you return to duty next morning, you are again caring for Mr Adams. Following handover at 07.30, you visit him and check his case notes. His volumetric pump has been discontinued and his fourth litre bag of intravenous fluid, 5% dextrose, is dripping at 28 drops per minute, via a macro giving set.

13 a How many ml/hour will 28 drops/minute deliver?
   b If approximately 300 ml have infused, when would you expect the bag to complete?

Following a visit from his medical officer, Mr Adams is told he can commence oral fluids. He is to begin with 50 ml of ice chips per hour for four hours.

14 What volume of fluid should be charted on the oral intake column of his fluid balance chart if he retains all of this fluid?

15 The Lomotil is reduced to 7.5 mg/day, to be given 8-hourly. Calculate his 14.00 dose.

16 At 15.00, Mr Adams can try some diluted apple juice. How much solute (apple juice) is required to make 200 ml of a 3 in 5 solution?

It is day three and you are following through with your care of Mr Adams. His intravenous infusion is now dripping at 15 drops per minute. The infusion line can be removed when this present bag completes.

17 If 135 ml remains in the bag, when would you expect it to complete?

18 Oral amoxycillin is to replace the intravenous route of administration. He is to have 2 g/day, to be given 6-hourly. How many mg should he receive in a single dose?

19 From available stock of 250 mg/capsule, how many capsules should you give him at 10.00?

20 Mr Adams is ready for discharge. He is to continue his antibiotics for a further four days. How many capsules would you expect the pharmacy to dispense?

 EXERCISE SEVEN

You are caring for Mr James, an elderly man who has been admitted to the ward with Diabetes, Congestive Cardiac Failure, and a leg ulcer. Following handover you visit him to give him his early morning medications.

1 His diuretic, oral frusemide, is due. He is to have 40 mg. If stock in the ward is 20 mg tablets, how many should he be given?

2   Following his breakfast, his oral hypoglycaemic medication, tolbutamide (Rastinon) is to be given. His order is for 500 mg. If stock in the ward is 1 g scored tablets, what should he be given?

His 10.00 medications are due and you are about to give them under the supervision of the registered nurse.

3   Oral Lanoxin 187.5 mcg has been ordered to slow and strengthen his heart beat. The only stock available in the ward is paediatric tablets, 62.5 mcg. How many tablets should you give him?

4   Oral nifedipine (Adalat) 20 mg is due. This medication decreases the workload of his heart and thus reduces his angina attacks. If stock on hand is equivalent to 0.01g, how many capsules should he receive?

5   Oral potassium chloride (Slow K) has been ordered to prevent hypokalaemia, a side effect of diuretic therapy. He is to have 0.6 g and stock in the ward is 600 mg tablets. How many should he be given?

Following his morning wash, you are to clean and redress his leg ulcer. During your assessment of this procedure, you ask him if he would like pain relief prior to beginning the dressing change. He tells you that he would like 'something as it usually hurts'.

6   He is permitted 20 mg of oral methadone (Physeptone) prior to his dressing changes. If stock in the ward is 10 mg tablets, how many should he be given?

7   He asks you to make up his diabetic cordial before you leave. He wants 1 L with a concentation of 30% cordial. How much cordial should you pour into the jug?

Assessment of his leg ulcer suggests that infection is present. The wound is seen by a medical officer who orders an antibiotic, ampicillin, 2 g per day, be given 6-hourly.

8   From available stock of 250 mg capsules, how many should you give him per dose?

Mr James is to have a fluid intake limit of 1.5 L per day. He insists on having five cups of tea (180 ml/cup) each day, and is emphatic that he cannot possibly sleep if he misses his bedtime hot chocolate (180 ml).

9 **a** How much fluid is available for other drinks?

   b Taking into account his medications, how could the remainder of his fluid be divided up so that it lasts all day?

   c Do you envisage any problems from his bedtime hot chocolate?

Next morning, you follow through with your care of Mr James. You visit him on the completion of handover to say hello and to check his case notes. He tells you that he 'feels awful', and you note that he has a rash on his trunk. He is seen by his doctor and his current antibiotics are discontinued.

10 A statim dose of the antihistamine promethazine hydrochloride (Phenergan) 20 mg is ordered, to be given intramuscularly. From stock on hand of 25 mg/ml, what volume should be drawn up?

11 The antibiotic oral cefaclor monohydrate (Ceclor) is ordered to replace the ampicillin. He is to have 750 mg each day, to be given 12-hourly. Calculate a single dose of this medication, and from available stock of 375 mg tablets, how many tablets should he be given at 08.00?

At 09.15 Mr James rings his bell to tell you that he is nauseated. By the time you reach him, he has vomited his breakfast. He has an order for intramuscular metoclopramide hydrochloride (Maxolon) 5 mg.

12 From available stock of 10 mg/2 ml, what volume should be drawn up?

13 At 10.00 an intravenous line is established. The 1 L of 0.9% sodium chloride is to last for 24 hours. How many ml/hour will need to be infused to fulfil this order, and if the drop factor for the giving set is 20 drops/ml, how fast should this infusion drip?

Following an evaluation of his electrolyte status, 1.5 g of potassium chloride (KCl) is to be added to the 1 L of 0.9% sodium chloride infusion, prior to its commencement.

14 **a** From available stock of 2 g/10 ml, what volume of potassium chloride should be drawn up?

    b What is the concentration, in mg/ml, of this KCl solution?
    c How many mg of KCl is Mr James receiving every hour?
    d What changes in Mr James's condition would indicate to you
        that he was developing hyperkalaemia?

Mr James's antibiotic order is changed once again as it is considered that the intravenous route is now more appropriate. He is to have cefoxitin sodium (Mefoxin) 3 g per day, to be given 6-hourly. This medication is available as 1 g of powder in a 10 ml vial, and manufacturing instructions indicate that the 1 g of powder will displace 1 ml of fluid when reconstituted.

15 **a** How many mg of cefoxitin sodium should he receive for his
       first dose?
   b If you are required to reconstitute this medication to a con-
       centration of 100 mg/ml, how much sterile water will you need
       to add to the 10 ml vial?
   c What volume of medication should you draw up for this dose?
   d This medication is to be added to the 22 ml of saline in the
       burette and infused over a 20-minute period. To what speed
       should you adjust the drip rate?

During a routine observation of Mr James later in the day, you note that he has developed dyspnoea and that his lips are cyanosed. You check his pulse and note that it is irregular and has risen from 76 to 98. His blood pressure has risen from 140/90 to 160/100. He is seen by a medical officer and ordered 40 mg of intravenous frusemide and 250 mcg of Lanoxin.

16 If frusemide is available as 10 mg/ml, what volume should be
    drawn up?

17 **a** Lanoxin stock in the ward is 0.5 mg/2 ml, how much should
       you draw up?
   b The Lanoxin is to be added to the remaining 10 ml of fluid in
       the burette and delivered over a 5-minute period. How fast
       should it drip?

Mr James becomes quite distressed and he tells you that 'he can't get any air into his lungs'. Oxygen is commenced and he is ordered 5 mg of intravenous morphine.

18 a If stock available is 10 mg/ml, what volume should he be given?

  b This is to be given as a bolus dose over four minutes. How should this be managed?

Mr James's condition begins to improve and he asks you to pour him half a glass of cordial. As you do so, you notice that he has a packet of Disprin capsules in his open locker drawer.

19 Does this medication have any significance in relation to any other medications he is taking? At 14.00 you measure his blood glucose level and the reading is 19.8 mmol/L. Sliding scale insulin is ordered, to be given according to the following format:

Under 7.9 mmol/L	nil
7.9 to 11.9	2 units of Actrapid
12 to 15.94 units	4 units
16 to 19.9	6 units
20 to 23.9	8 units
Above 24	notify the medical officer

20 For his reading of 19.8, how many units of insulin should he be given?

EXERCISE EIGHT

You are caring for Mr Bill Craven, a 74-year-old man who has been admitted to the ward with Pneumonia and chest pains. He has a past history of Chronic Renal Failure (CRF), Congestive Cardiac Failure (CCF), Hypertension, Angina and Dementia. On admission he is frail, unresponsive and dehydrated. An intravenous infusion has been established.

1 a The 1 L of normal saline is to infuse over a 24-hour period. How many ml/hour should this man receive, and if the drop factor for the giving set is 20 drops/ml, how fast should this infusion drip?

  b Considering that Mr Craven is dehydrated, why is the infusion rate set so low?

It is 07.30 and handover has just completed. While reviewing his case notes you note that his medications are due to be given.

2 Thiamine (Vitamin B₁) is given to help to reduce/lower the cholesterol level in his blood. From available stock of 50 mg tablets, how many tablets should he receive for his 100 mg dose?

3 Calcium carbonate (Caltrate) is given to support his poor dietary intake of calcium. 0.6 g is due and if the tablets available are 300 mg, what should he be given?

4 Amlodipine besylate is a medication to decrease myocardial contractility and in turn reduce oxygen demand. Mr Craven is to have 10 mg. If stock in the ward is 5 mg tablets, what should he be given?

5 Ranitidine, a medication which reduces the production of acid in the stomach, has been ordered. He is to have 150 mg. If stock available is 0.3 g scored tablets, what should you give him?

6 Atenolol, an anti-hypertensive, anti-angina medication is also required. Stock on hand is 25 mg tablets and he is to have 50 mg. What should you give him?

7 80 mg of the diuretic frusemide has been ordered. If stock is 40 mg tablets, what should he be given?

After his morning wash, he tells you that he 'aches all over'. You check his medication sheet and note that paracetamol 1 g may be given 6-hourly, PRN for pain. The registered nurse agrees that it should be given now.

8 If stock on hand is 500 mg tablets, how many tablets should you give to him?

At lunch time he refuses his meal, saying he 'feels sick'. His medication sheet indicates that metoclopramide (Maxolon) 10 mg may be given 4-hourly PRN. On checking his medications you note that nausea is a possible side effect of Ranitidine.

9 If Maxolon tablets on the ward are 5 mg each, how many tablets should you give him?

While doing your final medication check for the day you note that he is to have sertraline hydrochloride 50 mg each night. As you have not given this medication before, you look it up in 'MIMS' and note that it is an anti-depressant medication.

10 If ward stock is 100 mg scored tablets, what would you expect him to be given?

You are also caring for Mr Sam Grant, a 60-year-old man with a urinary tract infection following a kidney transplant. Mr Grant has a past history of Cerebrovascular Accident (CVA) and Transient Ischaemic Attacks (TIAs). His renal failure was secondary to Goodpasture's Syndrome. This was managed initially with Continuous Ambulatory Peritoneal Dialysis (CAPD) and replaced with haemodialysis two years ago. When you visit Mr Grant at 07.15 you note that an intravenous infusion is in progress and is dripping at 54 drops/minute.

11 a How many ml/hour is being delivered from the above order if a macro giving set is used?
   b How long would you expect this 1 L bag of 0.9% sodium chloride to last?

His 07.30 medications are due. Prednisolone 17.5 mg has been ordered. A second year nursing student is observing your care as it is her first day in the ward.

12 From available stock of 25 mg and 5 mg tablets, what should you give him?

13 The student asks why Mr Grant, who has a fairly severe urinary tract infection, is being given an anti-inflammatory medication. How should you respond to her question?

14 Asprin 100 mg is ordered to impede the clotting process as this man has a history of CVAs. If stock is equivalent to 0.1 g, what should he be given?

15 Ranitidine 150 mg is ordered to decrease gastric secretions (a side effect of prenisolone). From the available stock of 0.15 g, what should he be given?

16 At 10.00 mycophenolate mofetil (Cell Cept) 1.5 g is due. This medication provides prophylaxis against organ rejection and is given BD. Available stock is 500 mg tablets. How many tablets should he be given?

The transplant immuno-suppressive agent for this man is cyclosporin. The maintenance dose of this medication is 5 mg/kg/day, to be given BD.

17   **a**   If Mr Grant weighs 70 kg, what is his daily dose?
     b   How many mg should he receive for a single dose?
     c   From available stock of 100 mg, 50 mg, and 25 mg tablets, what should you give him?

18   At 12.00 his daily dose of 240 mg of intravenous gentamicin is due. Stock on the ward is an ampoule containing 80 mg/2 ml. What volume of gentamicin should be drawn up?

19   This medication is to be added to a 100 ml bag of 0.9% sodium chloride and infused via a secondary line over a one-hour period. To what speed (in drops/minute) should this line be adjusted if the drop factor for the giving set is 20 drops/ml?

At 12.00 you and the second year student are asked to go to lunch. The second year student is keen to change the intravenous when the current bag completes. You note that 90 ml remain in the bag and it is dripping at 50 drops/minute.

20   Have you both time for a 30-minute lunch break before the current bag completes?

EXERCISE NINE

Miss Fiona Reece is a 21-year-old woman who has been admitted to the Thoracic Medicine Unit with 'Exacerbation of Cystic Fibrosis'. On admission Fiona is febrile, her oxygen saturation level is 91%, she has a productive cough and is expectorating thick, green sputum. Her weight is 55 kg. Oxygen therapy is commenced and an infusion line is established.

1   **a**   The 1 L of 0.9% sodium chloride is dripping at 30 drops/minute with a drop factor of 20 drops/ml. How much intravenous fluid is she receiving every hour?
     b   How long would you expect this 1 L bag of fluid to last?

2   Fiona is to have a minimum of 200 ml of fluid every hour. Taking into account the amount she is receiving from the infusion, how much hourly fluid should you offer her as the oral contribution?

Antibiotics are commenced. Fiona is to have an initial dose of tobramycin sulphate 80 mg, which is to be added to the burette and infused over a 15-minute period.

3   **a**   If stock available is 0.04 g/ml, what volume should be drawn up?

    b   You add the prepared dose to the 20 ml of fluid in the burette. How fast will it need to drip to complete in the given time?

Because tobramycin sulphate can be quite toxic, Fiona's dose of this medication is now to be given routinely at a rate of 3 mg/kg of body weight/day, at 8-hourly intervals.

4   Calculate her daily dose and then a single dose of this medication. Results from her sputum culture will be unavailable for another 48 hours, so as a precautionary measure Fiona is to receive another antibiotic, ticarcillin sodium (Timentin), which is an extended spectrum penicillin. She is to have 200 mg/kg of body weight/day, to be given 6-hourly.

5   Calculate her daily dose and then a single dose of this medication.

This medication is available as 3 g of powder in a 15 ml vial and it is recommended (by the manufacturers) that an initial concentration of 200 mg/ml be achieved. Directions accompanying the medication instruct you to add 13 ml of sterile water to achieve the above concentration.

6   **a**   How many ml would be in the vial at this concentration following reconstitution?

    b   How much fluid has the 3 g of powder displaced?

    c   What volume should be drawn up for her first dose?

The medicated solution is to be added to an infusion line that is free from other medications, so a 50 ml bag of 0.9% sodium chloride is used as a secondary line, with the main infusion turned off. The drop factor for this giving set is 20 drops/ml.

7 Taking into account the medication you will add to this bag, calculate the rate of flow for the Timentin in the 0.9% sodium chloride, if it is to infuse over a 30-minute period.

Fiona says that she feels nauseated. She has an order for oral metoclopramide hydrochloride (Maxolon) and she may have 10 mg 6-hourly PRN.

8 From available stock of 0.01 mg per tablet, what should she be given?

9 a A Heparin flush of 500 units is ordered 6-hourly. From stock in the ward of 5000 units/ml, what volume of Heparin should be drawn up?

   b With accuracy of dose in mind, what sort of a syringe should be used to draw up this medication?

   c The Heparin flush is to be delivered at a concentration of 100 units of Heparin per ml, so how much sterile water is required to achieve this concentration?

   d Explain how this task could be achieved, taking into account the volume of Heparin required.

10 a Fiona is ordered ranitidine hydrochloride 150 mg BD to inhibit gastric secretions. Stock on hand is 300 mg scored tablets. What should you give her?

    b Does this medication have any undesirable side effects related to the gastro-intestinal tract?

11 The second dose of tobramycin is due. With reference to Q 4 for dose and Q 3 for stock available, calculate the volume to be drawn up.

When you arrive on duty next afternoon, you continue to care for Fiona. Her intravenous solution of 5% dextrose is dripping at 25 drops/minute. You check her fluid order for the day and note that this 1 L bag is to last for ten hours as her oral intake is less than what was planned.

12 Is the current rate of flow correct? If not, to what rate of flow will you need to adjust the set to maintain the given order?

13 Fiona asks for 'something for a headache'. She is permitted 1 g of paracetamol. If stock in the ward is 500 mg tablets, what should she be given?

14 A salbutamol (Ventolin) inhalation is to be given to reduce bronchospasm. She is to have 5 mg at a 1 to 1 ratio with sterile normal saline. Stock in the ward is 5 mg/ml. How much saline is required for this task?

At 17.00 you are to give Fiona her Viokase tablets. These tablets contain the pancreatic enzymes needed to assist in the digestion of food. She is to have 0.975 g/day, in three equally divided doses. Stock available is 325 mg tablets.

15 How many tablets should you give her now?

Following her meal, she vomits 300 ml of undigested food. Intravenous metoclopramide 7.5 mg is ordered, to be given by slow injection. Stock in the ward is 10 mg/2 ml.

16 a What volume should be drawn up for the 7.5 mg dose?
  b How many ml/minute would you need to infuse to give this dose over a 2-minute period?
  c Is Fiona currently receiving any medications which could cause nausea or vomiting?

17 To assist Fiona to sleep, Temazepam 20 mg has been ordered. Tablets in the ward are 10 mg, so what should she be given?

When you return to duty after two days off, you visit Fiona at 07.30. She tells you that she is feeling better and asks you to dilute her orange and mango juice for her as it is too sweet.

18 How much water is required to make up 300 ml of a 4 to 1 solution of fruit juice?

19 Her intravenous infusion is dripping at 25 drops per minute and 360 ml remain. How much fluid is she receiving every hour?

At 10.00 you are to add her antibiotic (refer to Q 6c for the amount) to the remaining 46 ml of fluid in the burette. On completion of this medication administration, Fiona may be discharged. She asks you to telephone her family to collect her and take her home.

20 **a** When the medication is added, what volume of fluid is in the burette?

   b If it drips at 30 drops per minute, when will it complete?

   c At what time would you arrange for her family to collect her?

EXERCISE TEN

Hamilton Collier is a young man on holiday in this country. He has been admitted to hospital with severe Asthma and a chest infection. On admission his breathing is laboured and noisy, his colour is cyanosed, he is febrile and dehydrated. His weight is 60 kg. Oxygen therapy is commenced and an intravenous line is established.

1 **a** He is ordered a loading dose of intravenous aminophylline (a bronchodilator) 200 mg. Stock available is 0.25 g/10 ml. Calculate the volume to be given.

   b Following this medication, which was given in a hurry, he complains of dizziness and palpitations. You take his blood pressure and note that he is hypotensive. What is the physiological reason for his present condition?

   c How could this condition have been possibly avoided?

He has with him an antibiotic prescription for his chest infection and the medical officer agrees to continue with this medication. This prescription states that he is to have cefoxitin sodium (Mefoxin) 25 mg/pound of body weight/day, to be given 6-hourly.

2 Remembering that there are 2.2 pounds per kg, convert his weight to pounds.

3 What is the daily dose of medication that Hamilton has been ordered, and how many mg should he have for a single dose?

Mefoxin is available as 1 gram of powder in a 10 ml vial for reconstitution. Instructions indicate that the 1 gram of powder will displace 0.5 ml of fluid when a solution is formed.

4 How much sterile water is required to create a solution with a concentration of 200 mg/ml, and what volume of fluid should be drawn up for his first dose of this medication?

The medicated solution that you have just drawn up is to be added to a 50 ml bag of 0.9% sodium chloride and delivered (via a secondary line) over a 30-minute period.

5 How fast should this medicated infusion drip if the drop factor for the giving set is 20 drops/ml?

A maintenance dose of aminophylline has been ordered. 360 mg is to be added to the current 1 L of 0.9% sodium chloride. Stock available is 250 mg/10 ml ampoule and this medication is to infuse at the rate of 10 mcg/kg of body weight/minute.

6 **a** What volume of aminophylline should be drawn up for this order?
   b What is the concentration (in mcg/ml) of this medicated infusion?
   c How fast should the volumetric infusion pump be set to deliver the above order?

Hamilton asks for his Mucomyst inhalant as he is having difficulty expectorating the viscous mucus secretions. The label on the bottle states that it is a 20% solution of Acetylcysteine. He asks you to prepare 3 ml of a 10% solution for his nebulizer.

7 What should you actually put into the nebulizer?

He is to have a salbutamol (Ventolin) inhalation every four hours. Stock available is a 0.5% solution which is to be given at a 1 to 1 ratio with 0.9% sodium chloride.

8 If the total volume of this inhalation is 2 ml, what volume is actually Ventolin?

Next morning when you come on duty Hamilton's condition has markedly improved. He tells you that his breathing is much easier and his chest feels less constricted. His intravenous aminophylline has completed and he is to have oral theophylline (Elixophyllin) 5 mg/kg of body weight/day, to be given 8-hourly.

9 **a** What is his daily dose of this medication?
   b Stock available is a 500 ml bottle with a concentration of 80 mg/15 ml. Calculate the volume of medication you should pour for him per dose.

10 Hamilton is commenced on oral prednisolone to reduce the inflammatory response in his respiratory system. He is to have 30 mg/day for the next 48 hours. This medication is to be given 4-hourly. If stock available is 5 mg scored tablets, how many should you give for a single dose?

11 His intravenous therapy is continuing and the present bag of 5% dextrose is to infuse at the rate of 80 ml/hour. How long would you expect this 1 L bag to last and how fast should it be dripping?

12 Hamilton is now up and about. His prednisolone has been reduced to 20 mg/day, to be given 6-hourly. With reference to Q 10 for stock available, how many tablets per dose should he receive now?

13 You are to encourage oral hydration. He asks you to dilute a 600 ml carton of apricot juice to a ratio of 6 in 10. How much iced water will you need to add?

14 It is day four and Hamilton can go home when his intravenous antibiotic completes. 70 ml remain in the bag and it is dripping at the rate of 35 drops/minute. When should you ask his taxi to call for him?

Mrs Lobinski has been admitted to the ward with Pulmonary Oedema. She is wheezy, has dyspnoea, is anxious, apprehensive and restless.

15 She has been ordered 12 mg of morphine to reduce her pain and anxiety. If stock available is 15 mg/ml, what volume should you draw up?

An intravenous line is inserted and 0.5 L of 0.9% sodium chloride is dripping at the rate of 30 drops/minute via a micro giving set with a drop factor of 60 drops/ml.

16 How much fluid is she receiving every hour and how long would you expect this bag to last?

17 The diuretic frusemide 60 mg is to be given immediately intra-venously. Stock on hand is equivalent to 0.05 g/5 ml. Calculate the volume to be drawn up.

18 Intravenous digoxin has been ordered to slow and strengthen the heart beat. She is to have this for the next 24 hours. Mrs Lobinski, who weighs 60 kg, is to have 20 mcg/kg of body weight/day, to be given 6-hourly. What is her daily dose of digoxin?

19 From available stock of 0.5 mg/ml, what volume should be drawn up for a single dose?

20 This medication is to be added to 20 ml of fluid in the paediatric burette and infused over a 30-minute period. How fast should this medicated solution drip?

 ANSWERS

EXERCISE ONE

1 15.75 ml/hour

2 24 ml/hour

3 3 ml/hour

4 10 ml/hour

5 117 ml/hour

6 25 ml/hour

7 5 ml/hour

8 40 ml/hour

9 33.33 ml/hour

10 **a** 10 g + 90 ml   **b** 25 g + 75 ml   **c** 30 g + 70 ml
    d 50 g + 50 ml

11 **a** 50 g + 200 ml   **b** 25 g + 225 ml   **c** 100 g + 150 ml
    d 75 g + 175 ml

12 9 grams

13 10 grams

14 90 ml

15 180 ml/hour

16 10 ml

17 10 ml

18 **a** 5 mg/ml   **b** 4 ml/hour

19 **a** 3 mg/minute **b** 0.6 ml
    c 36 ml/hour for 4 minutes only

20 **a** 100 ml/hour **b** 125 ml/hour **c** 100 ml/hour
    d 50 ml/hour   **e** 50 ml/hour

EXERCISE TWO

1   1 × 150 mg + 1 × 300 mg capsules

2   **a** 200 mg/day   **b** 1/2 tablet

3   1/2 tablet

4   2 tablets

5   1/2 tablet

6   20%

7   9000 kilojoules

8   13.33% will be protein

9   68 grams of fat/day

10 5280 kilojoules

11 198 grams of complex carbohydrates

12 2112 kilojoules for simple sugars

13 5 hours

14 67 drops/minute

15 83 drops/minute

16 **a** 11.25 ml   **b** In approximately 4 hours at 15.30
    c 40 drops/minute

17 **a** 2 ml/dose   **b** 44 drops/minute

18 1 tablet/dose

19 60 ml of solvent

20 10 days

EXERCISE THREE

1 80 drops/minute

2 **a** 50 kg   **b** 3 grams/day   **c** 750 mg/dose

3 **a** 9 ml   **b** 7.5 ml

4 36 drops/minute

5 1.4 ml

6 **a** 40 drops/minute   **b** 6 hours 20 minutes

7 **a** Aspirin is an antipyretic medication to help reduce his fever.
   b 60 ml of water

8 12 ml/dose

9 Approximately 125 ml every 2 hours

10 1 in 5

11 As an intravenous drug user, Paul's tolerance is probably altered.

12 2 ml

13 56 drops/minute

14 2 ml

15 4 mcg/ml

16 100 ml/hour

17 2 capsules

18 6 ml

19 $1\frac{1}{2}$ hours

20 28 capsules

EXERCISE FOUR

1 2 tablets

2 56 drops/minute

3 2 ml

4 0.8 ml

5 Yes, it is on schedule

6 125 ml/hour

7 **a** 4 ml   **b** 56 ml   **c** 1 mg/ml   **d** 2.5 ml/hour

8 1 ml

9 Yes (62 kg × 0.5/kg = 31)

10 **a** 9 ml of sterile water   **b** 750 mg/dose
    c 7.5 ml/dose   **d** 37 drops/minute

11 1 × 120 mg tablet/dose

12 Yes (3000 ml ÷ 24 hours)

13 120 ml

14 **a** 1 mg/minute   **b** 1 ml/minute
    c 60 ml/hour for 3 minutes

15 33 drops/minute

16 50 grams/L

17 800 kilojoules

18 0.16 ml or 16 units on an insulin syringe

19 $1\frac{1}{2}$ tablets

20 2 capsules/dose

EXERCISE FIVE

1 2 tablets

2 2 tablets/hour

3 **a** 16 tablets **b** 8 grams

4 5 hours, 67 drops/minute

5 Intake 4000 ml, output 3600 ml

6 1.5 ml

7 0.8 ml

8 Yes, you have just 30 minutes before the bag completes.

9 **a** 1.5 hours **b** 40 drops/minute

10 **a** 8 ml **b** 108 ml **c** 4.5 ml/hour
   d 3.7 mg/ml **e** 66.6 mg/4 hours **f** Yes

11 1.5 ml

12 **a** 1 ml/minute **b** 3.7 mg/ml **c** 14.8 mg of pethidine

13 **a** 4.1 ml **b** 82.5 ml **c** 55 drops/minute

14 **a** 13.3 ml **b** 1 mg/ml
   c 125 ml/hour and 42 drops/minute
   d Observe her for hyperkalaemia

15 **a** A minimum of 30 ml/hour or 45 ml in $1\frac{1}{2}$ hours
   b No, it should be 42 drops/minute
   c Yes
   d Notify charge nurse or medical officer in charge

16 **a** To remove the KCl from the line
   b Packed cells are given for anaemia whereas whole blood is given following a haemorrhage
   c To note any reaction, so that the infusion can be stopped immediately to minimise harm to the client
   d 50 drops/minute

17 **a** If dextrose follows blood, aggregation of red blood cells could occur.
   b 67 drops/minute **c** 33 drops/minute

18 **a** Bowel sounds would be present **b** 120 ml

19 100 ml of ice water

20 2 ml

EXERCISE SIX

1 9 stone 6 pounds

2 3.636 L

3 333 ml/hour

4 167 ml/hour

5 83 ml/hour

6 **a** 30 mg/day, 7.5 mg/dose   **b** 1.5 ml/dose

7 **a** 5 ml   **b** 5 ml

8 55 drops/minute

9 6.7 ml

10 $5\frac{1}{2}$ hours, 19 drops/minute

11 **a** Give one dose immediately   **b** 0.8 ml

12 5 mg/dose and 2 tablets/dose

13 **a** 84 ml/hour   **b** In 8 hours 20 minutes or at 15.50

14 200 ml

15 1 tablet

16 120 ml

17 In 3 hours

18 500 mg/dose

19 2 capsules

20 32 capsules

EXERCISE SEVEN

1 2 tablets

2 1/2 tablet

3 3 tablets

4 2 capsules

5 1 tablet

6 2 tablets

7 300 ml

8 2 capsules

9 **a** 420 ml   **b** Allow 100 ml for each medication administration.
   c No, as he's been having hot chocolate as his usual bedtime drink, it's probably not harmful to him. Sweeten it with an artificial sweetener.

10 0.8 ml

11 1 tablet/dose

12 1 ml

13 42 ml/hour, 14 drops/minute

14 **a** 7.5 ml   **b** 1.5 mg/ml   **c** 62.5 mg/hour
   d A change in cardiac status, general weakness

15 **a** 750 mg/dose   **b** 9 ml   **c** 7.5 ml
   d 30 drops/minute

16 4 ml

17 **a** 1 ml   **b** 44 drops/minute

18 **a** 0.5 ml   **b** 1 mg statim and then every minute until the medication is infused

19 Salicylates may potentiate the hypoglycaemic action of Rastinon.

20 6 units

EXERCISE EIGHT

1 **a** 42 ml/hour, 14 drops/minute
   b He has a history of CCF & CRF so it is important to not cause circulatory overload.

2 2 tablets

3 2 tablets

4 2 tablets

5 1/2 tablet

6 2 tablets

7 2 tablets

8 2 tablets

9 2 tablets

10 1/2 tablet

11 **a** 162 ml/hour **b** Approximately 6 hours 10 mins

12 1/2 × 25 mg + 1 × 5 mg tablets

13 It is part of his immuno-suppressive therapy following his kidney transplant.

14 1 tablet

15 1 tablet

16 3 tablets

17 **a** 350 mg **b** 175 mg
      c 1 × 100 mg, 1 × 50 mg, 1 × 25 mg tablets

18 6 ml

19 35 drops/minute

20 Yes, this infusion should last 36 minutes

EXERCISE NINE

1 **a** 90 ml/hour **b** Approximately 11 hours

2 110 ml/hour

3 **a** 2 ml **b** 29 drops/minute

4 165 mg/day & 55 mg/dose

5 11 000 mg/day & 2750 mg/dose

6 **a** 15 ml **b** 2 ml **c** 13.75 ml

7 42–43 drops/minute

8 1 tablet

9 **a** 0.1 ml **b** An insulin syringe **c** 5 ml
  d Open a 5 ml ampoule of sterile water, add the 0.1 ml of
  Heparin, mix with syringe and draw it all up.

10 **a** 1/2 tablet **b** It has the potential to cause nausea in
  some clients.

11 1.375 or 1.4 ml

12 No, it should be dripping at 33 drops/minute

13 2 tablets

14 1 ml

15 1 tablet

16 **a** 1.5 ml
  b 0.5 ml statim, then repeat after 1 and 2 minutes
  c Zantac has the potential to cause nausea

17 2 tablets

18 60 ml of water

19 75 ml/hour

20 **a** 59.75 ml **b** Approximately 40 minutes
  c 11.00

EXERCISE TEN

1 **a** 8 ml
  b Aminophylline causes direct central nervous system and
  cardiovascular stimulation if given rapidly.
  c It should be given by slow intravenous infusion.

2 132 pounds

3 3300 mg/day, 825/dose

4 4.5 ml should be added, draw up 4.1 ml

5   36 drops/minute

6   **a**   14.4 ml   **b**   360 mcg/ml
    c   Dose (in mcg) × Weight (in kg) × 60 (mins/hr) ÷ dose (mcg)
    in solution = 100ml/hour

7   1.5 ml of Mucomyst & 1.5 ml of sterile normal saline

8   1 ml

9   **a**   300 mg   **b**   18.75 ml

10   1 tablet/dose

11   It should drip at 27 drops/minute and last for 12.5 hours

12   1 tablet/dose

13   400 ml of iced water

14   In approximately 45 minutes

15   0.8 ml

16   30 ml/hour and 16 hours 40 minutes

17   6 ml

18   1200 mcg or 1.2 mg

19   0.6 ml

20   40 drops/minute

6

Complex Calculations

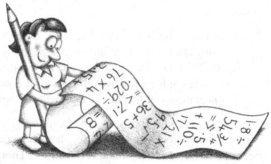

Objectives

At the completion of the following exercises it is expected that the student should be able to use nursing calculations with speed and accuracy in relation to:

- the metric system

- oral, parenteral and intravenous medications

- intravenous therapy, including volumetric pumps

EXERCISE ONE

Mrs Shirley Robbins is a young woman who is admitted to the Oncology Unit on Monday afternoon for a Wertheim's hysterectomy at 08.30 on Wednesday, following a diagnosis of stage III carcinoma of the cervix. She weighs 50 kg. Because the extent of the cancerous invasion is unclear, the surgeon has ordered that a bowel preparation be carried out prior to surgery. A diet low in fibre is commenced to reduce the faecal content in the bowel. Mrs Robbins, who is 32 years old and has two young children, is very anxious and distressed about her prognosis. You have been assigned to care for her during her hospital stay.

1   Diazepam 2 mg has been ordered to reduce her anxiety, and it is to be given nocte for the next two nights. If stock in the ward is 1 mg tablets, how many tablets/dose should she be given?

At 08.00 on Tuesday, she is commenced on an antibiotic regime for 24 hours to reduce the microbial population in her bowel. She is to have neomycin sulphate (Neosulf), which is available as 500 mg scored tablets.

2   a   Initially, she is to have 1 g every hour for four hours. How many tablets/dose should she be given?
    b   At the end of the four hours she is to continue this medication, having 1 g for a further four doses, at 4-hourly intervals. How many grams of this medication will she have in total?

At 14.00 she is commenced on a medication to cleanse her bowel. She is now advised to have a low-fibre diet and nourishing fluids until twelve hours before her operation. An intravenous line is established to ensure that dehydration does not occur, and to begin with, 1 L of 0.9% sodium chloride is to infuse at the rate of 0.2 L/hour.

3   a   If the giving set emits 20 drops/ml, to what rate of flow, in drops/minute, should the set be regulated, and when could you expect this bag to complete?
    b   While receiving the medication to cleanse her bowel, Mrs Robbins has the potential to lose quite a lot of fluid. Apart from sodium, which is being replaced, what other electrolyte could be lost in excessive amounts?

c What observations of Mrs Robbins would indicate to you that she was suffering an excessive loss of the electrolyte mentioned in the previous question?

While attending to Mrs Robbins she confides in you her concerns. She asks you, 'What are my chances of surviving this disease?' You are aware that approximately 1000 new cases of cervical cancer were diagnosed in Australia this year and that around 350 women will die from this disease.

4 **a** What are her odds for survival?

   b If 70% (that is, 350 women) of all uterine cancers begin in the cervix, what is the approximate overall death rate from uterine cancer in Australia per year?

It is the policy of the operating surgeon that all hysterectomies have a vaginal douche prior to the operation and at 18.00 you are asked to perform this task. A 1.5% Betadine solution is to be used.

5 How much pure Betadine is required to make up 1 L of solution using warm tap water as the solvent?

It is 07.20 on Wednesday morning, and you have just completed Mrs Robbins's bowel washout. You used 5 L of warm tap water for this assignment and on completion of the task, you note that the return measures 4.7 L.

6 What should be charted on the intake and output columns of her fluid balance chart and what has happened to the remainder of the fluid that you infused into the bowel?

Her pre-operative check list has just been completed and you are ready to administer her premedication. She is to have 70 mg of pethidine and 600 mcg of Atropine. She asks you why she has to have an injection now, as she is not in any pain.

7 **a** Explain to her the purpose of the premedication.

   b From available stock of 100 mg/2 ml, what volume of pethidine should be drawn up?

   c Atropine is available in a one ml ampoule with a concentration of 0.6 mg/ml. What volume should you draw up?

At 08.10 you commence her next intravenous fluid order. She is to have 1 L of 5% dextrose over a 4-hour period.

8 What volume per hour will she receive and how fast should this infusion order drip?

At 12.30 Mrs Robbins returns to the ward from Recovery, following the removal of her uterus, fallopian tubes and ovaries. Her infusion is continuing and it has a 'secondary line' for pain relief; she has an indwelling catheter in situ, a vaginal pack in place and a negative pressure drain in the lower right side of her vertical abdominal incision. You observe in her case notes that two units of blood have been ordered.

9 1 L of 0.9% sodium chloride was commenced at 12.20 and is dripping at 40 drops/minute. How many ml/hour will this infusion deliver?

10 Her urinary catheter was inserted at 11.30 and the drainage bag has 60 ml of fluid in it. How many ml/hour would you expect this post-operative woman to excrete, as a minimum?

The secondary line mentioned above contains a medicated solution of 300 mg of pethidine in 100 ml of 0.9% sodium chloride and it is to last for 20 hours.

11 **a** What is the concentration (in mg/ml) of this medicated solution?
    b How many ml/hour would you expect the infusion pump to be delivering?
    c How many mg of pethidine per hour is Mrs Robbins receiving from this order?
    d Is the dose she is receiving within normal limits for a client weighing 50 kg, if the MIMS (2002) recommends that the maximum desirable dose of intravenous pethidine for a person of Mrs Robbins's size and age should be 50 mg 3-hourly?
    e What is probably the most important side effect that you should monitor while the pethidine infusion is in progress?

The registered nurse asks you to give Mrs Robbins her intravenous antibiotic, which is being given as a surgical prophylaxis. She is to have cephalothin sodium (Keflin Neutral) 750 mg 6-hourly. This medication is available as 1 g of powder in a 10 ml vial for reconstitution.

12 **a** Instructions accompanying this medication indicate that you are to add 2 ml of sterile water to achieve a concentration of

500 mg/2.2 ml. How much fluid has this 1 g of powder dis-placed when reconstitution occurred?

b What volume of medication should be drawn up for her first dose?

c You are to add this medication to 20 ml of fluid in the burette and infuse it over a 10-minute period. How fast should it drip?

Mrs Robbins complains of nausea. You check her medication sheet and note that intravenous metoclopramide 0.5 mg/kg/day has been ordered. This medication may be given 4-hourly PRN. Stock available is 5 mg/ml.

13 a What volume of medication should be drawn up for this dose?

b If this medication is to be infused over a 4-minute period, how should you proceed?

Mrs Robbins calls you and tells you that her pain is unbearable. You report this information to the registered nurse and you are asked to give her a bolus dose of 12 mg of pethidine over a 4-minute period. She will supervise you fulfilling this task.

14 a How many mg/minute should Mrs Robbins receive from this order?

b What volume of fluid contains the above dose/minute?

c To what speed (in ml/hour) should you adjust the infusion pump to accommodate this order?

d As soon as the order has completed, what observations should you make of the apparatus and the client?

When you return to duty next morning, you visit Mrs Robbins. As you chat with her, you note that her intravenous infusion is dripping faster than you would have expected. At 07.30 you check her medication order and note that this 1 L of 5% dextrose was commenced at 05.00 and is to last for ten hours.

15 a If it is dripping at 50 drops/minute, how many ml/hour is she currently receiving?

b If the order is for this bag to last for ten hours, how fast should it be dripping?

c You note that 700 ml of fluid remain in the bag. When could you expect this bag to complete following your adjustment to the correct rate of flow?

At 10.30 her blood arrives in the ward and the registered nurse asks you to remove the bag of 5% dextrose and replace it with a 100 ml bag of 0.9% sodium chloride.

16 a How much fluid would you expect to see charted on the fluid balance chart in relation to the bag of 5% dextrose which you are removing?

b Why have you been asked to replace the dextrose with 0.9% sodium chloride?

c If the 100 ml of 0.9% sodium chloride is to infuse over a 30-minute period, how fast should it drip?

At 11.00 the blood is commenced and each unit of 400 ml is to last for four hours. You have been asked to commence each unit at the rate of 45 ml/hour for the first fifteen minutes.

17 a How fast should the blood drip for the first fifteen minutes?

b Why have you been asked to commence the infusion of blood at such a slow rate of flow?

c To what speed, in drops/minute, will the blood need to drip if 0.4 L is to complete in four hours?

It is day three post-operation and you are to assist Mrs Robbins to shower this morning. She asks if she can wait until her infusion completes as it can be removed on completion of this bag. You note that 90 ml remain in the bag and it is dripping at 20 drops/minute.

18 a How many ml/hour is 20 drops/minute delivering?

b If it is 08.15, at what time could you expect to return to shower Mrs Robbins?

Following her shower, Mrs Robbins asks for 'something for her pain'. On checking her medication order you note that she can have 45 mg of codeine phosphate, 6-hourly PRN for pain relief.

19 If stock on hand is 30 mg tablets, what should you give her?

20 What is a common side effect of the above medication that could be enhanced by Mrs Robbins's current lack of appetite and decreased mobility, and what advice could she be given to reduce the effects of this medication?

EXERCISE TWO

Mr Saul Jacobs is a 58-year-old man who has been admitted to the cardiac ward with severe chest pain which was not relieved by his usual medication, Anginine. He states that he took 1 ½ tablets (0.6 mg/tablet) and his pain is still quite severe. He has a history of a myocardial infarction two years ago, and has had two episodes of Congestive Cardiac Failure (CCF) since then. On admission he was ordered morphine sulphate, 200 mcg/kg of body weight for pain, and his wife tells you that he weighs 70 kg.

1 Write the dose of Anginine that he took in mcg and mg.

2 a Calculate the dose of morphine he should be given.
   b If stock available is 15 mg/ml, what volume should be drawn up for this dose?
   c What type of syringe would be most suitable for the administration of this dose of morphine?

It is 12.15 and an intravenous infusion is established to maintain hydration and to create a port of entry for any emergencies. 1 L of 0.9% sodium chloride is to infuse at the rate of 25 drops/minute, via a drop factor of 20 drops/ml.

3 a How many ml/hour will he receive from this infusion?
   b How long would you expect this infusion to last?
   c Taking into account his previous history of CCF, would you consider his fluid intake to be acceptable?

He is to continue with his usual dose of digoxin, a medication that slows the heart rate and increases the force of its contractions. He is to have 0.25 mg daily, to be given BD.

4 From available ward stock of 125 mcg tablets, what should he be given for his morning dose of this medication?

At midday he refuses his meal, saying he feels nauseated and has a headache. His medical officer visits him and he is ordered metoclopramide, 0.5 mg/kg of body weight/day, to be given 6-hourly PRN.

5 Calculate a single dose of this medication if stock on hand is 5 mg/ml, and state the volume which should be drawn up for his first dose.

At 14.00 he rings his bell and tells you that he feels very breathless. You note that he has severe dyspnoea, frothy, blood-stained sputum and is cyanosed. His medical officer is called and orders intravenous frusemide, 80 mg.

6 If available stock is equivalent to 0.01 g/ml, what volume of medication should be drawn up?

At 15.00 Mr Jacobs asks to be helped out onto the commode. He is found several minutes later slumped half off his chair and not responding to stimuli. He is returned to bed, oxygen is commenced and the resuscitation team is called. When the team arrives, you are asked to draw up 100 mg of lignocaine hydrochloride as part of the resuscitation process.

7 Lignocaine suppresses ventricular arrhythmia. If stock of Lignocaine is 20 mg/ml, in a 5 ml vial, what volume should be drawn up?

8 The Lignocaine is to be followed by 0.6 mg of Atropine to treat sinus bradycardia and associated hypotension as well as increased ventricular irritability. From available stock of 600 mcg/ml, what volume should be drawn up?

Mr Jacob's recovery is somewhat hesitant. He is commenced on a Lignocaine infusion of 2 grams of Lignocaine in 500 ml of 0.9% sodium chloride.

9 **a** To what speed, in ml/hour, should the volumetric pump be set if he is to have 4 mg of Lignocaine per minute for the first hour?
   b During the second hour, this infusion is to be reduced to 40 ml/hour. How many mg/hour will he receive from this order?
   c This infusion is to continue at the rate of 120 mg/hour on completion of the second hour. How many ml/hour will deliver this maintenance dose?

Following further investigations, Mr Jacobs is given a provisional diagnosis of Myocardial Infarction. He slowly recovers but is extremely anxious. He is ordered intravenous diazepam, 8 mg, to be given statim, at the rate of 1 mg/minute. Stock in the ward is 10 mg/2 ml.

10 a What volume should be drawn up and given?

   b Why does this intravenous medication need to be injected slowly?

   c Is there any reason why this medication cannot be added to a secondary line and infused slowly?

11 2.5 mg of intravenous morphine is to be given to control pain. Stock on hand is 10 mg/ml. Using an insulin syringe, what volume should be drawn up?

Alteplase (Actilyse) is ordered. This medication binds to fibrin in a thrombus and converts the entrapped plasminogen to plasmin, thus initiating local fibrinolysis with minimal systemic effects. This medication is to be given in three stages: first an initial intravenous bolus dose of 15 mg is given, followed by 0.75 mg/kg over 30 minutes and completed with 0.5 mg/kg over 60 minutes.

12 Stock available is 50 mg of powder, to be combined with 50 ml of accompanying solvent. Following reconstitution, what volume should be drawn up and given for the initial bolus dose?

The bolus dose of alteplase is to be followed by a 30-minute infusion of this medication at the rate of 0.75 mg/kg of body weight.

13 a How many mg of alteplase is required for this phase of his treatment?

   b Taking into account that the concentration of this medication (following reconstitution) is 1 mg/ml, to what speed (in ml/hour) will the infusion pump need to be set?

On completion of the above quantity of alteplase, the dosage is reduced to 0.5 mg/kg of body weight, which is to infuse over a 60-minute period.

14 a State this dose in mg.

   b State the volume per hour that needs to be infused to deliver this phase of the order.

Next day when you return to duty, you are again assigned to care for Mr Jacobs. You visit him after handover and note that an intravenous infusion is still in progress, and a secondary line containing Heparin, 40 000 units in 0.25 L 0.9% sodium chloride, is attached. He tells you that he feels better but is very tired. He is to remain in bed for the time being.

15 **a** His infusion of 1 L of 5% dextrose is dripping at 45 drops per minute. How much fluid will this infusion deliver to him each hour if the drop factor for this giving set is 60 drops/ml?

   b How long would you expect this infusion to last?

   c If it commenced at 04.00 this morning, at what time would you expect it to complete?

16 **a** The secondary line attached for the Heparin infusion is to deliver 1600 units of Heparin per hour. To what speed, in ml/hour, should the infusion pump be set to deliver the ordered dose?

   b What is the concentration, in units/ml, of this medicated solution?

   c How long should this infusion last?

   d How much fluid is Mr Jacobs receiving from these two infusions every hour?

Mr Jacobs remains nauseated and so his routine medications of oral digoxin and frusemide are to be given intravenously for the time being.

17 Digoxin 125 mcg is to be given and if stock on the ward is 500 mcg/2 ml, calculate the volume to be drawn up for his morning dose.

18 Intravenous frusemide 15 mg is to be given daily. Stock is 20 mg/2 ml. What volume should be given?

It is day three post-infarction and Mr Jacobs is permitted to sit out of bed today. He is tolerating food and fluids and so his intravenous has been discontinued.

19 **a** Heparin has been replaced with warfarin sodium (Coumadin) tablets. A dose of 6 mg/day has been ordered, to be given BD. How many mg/dose should he have?

   b From available stock of 2 mg scored tablets, what should he be given each dose?

When you take his blood pressure at 10.30, he tells you he has just had 'a couple of aspirins for his headache'.

20 **a** Is there any significance in this statement in relation to his current medications?

b How will you manage this knowledge that you have just acquired?

 EXERCISE THREE

Mr Terry Nutzon is a 63-year-old man who has been admitted to the cardiac ward with Acute Heart Failure. He has a past history of Coronary Artery Disease and is hypertensive, orthopnoeac and cyanotic on admission. He is placed in a high Fowler's position, oxygen is commenced, and an intravenous infusion is established to maintain an open line should medications be needed in an emergency. On admission his weight is 75 kg.

1 His wife, who is observing your admission process, notes his weight and tells you that he is normally 11 stone 4 pounds. Remembering that 1 stone equals 14 pounds and that 2.2 pounds equal 1 kg, what is the difference between his usual weight and now?

2 Approximately how much extra fluid is he currently retaining?

3 Intravenous frusemide 80 mg is to be given immediately and then 6/24, to reduce his circulatory overload. Stock on the ward is 5 ml ampoules with a concentration of 10 mg/ml. What volume should he be given?

4 A statim dose of 15 mg of subcutaneous morphine has been ordered to reduce his anxiety and discomfort. If stock on the ward is 10 mg/ml, what volume should be drawn up?

Intravenous digoxin is to be given to slow and strengthen cardiac contractions. During the next 24 hours he is to have 1 mg in two equally divided doses.

5 From available stock of 500 mcg/2 ml, what volume/dose should be drawn up?

6 **a** The intravenous infusion of 0.5 L of 5% dextrose is dripping at the rate of 40 drops per minute via a micro-dropper. What

volume of dextrose is he receiving each hour from this infusion? State the purpose of using a micro-dropper for this client.

b How long would you expect this infusion to last?

During the admission process, you take and record Mr Nutzon's blood pressure. It is 210/130, so you report this to the registered nurse who alerts the physician. Sodium nitroprusside is to be added to his infusion, to relax smooth muscle thus allowing dilation of peripheral blood vessels. The registered nurse asks you to make up a solution, under her guidance, with a concentration of 100 mcg/ml. The Nitroprusside is to be added to the 500 ml of 5% dextrose which has just commenced.

7 How many mg of sodium nitroprusside are required to make up the ordered concentration?

8 How will the dilation of peripheral blood vessels assist in reducing his elevated blood pressure?

You have reconstituted the sodium nitroprusside powder with 2 ml of 5% dextrose (the only compatible solution as stated in the manufacturer's instructions), and added it to the 0.5 L bag of 5% dextrose currently infusing, and you have placed an aluminium foil wrap around the bag as instructed.

9 State the purpose of the aluminium foil wrap around the solution.

The initial rate of flow for this infusion is 0.5 mcg/kg of body weight/minute. A volumetric pump is attached to the line to ensure an accurate delivery.

10 What volume per hour will deliver the above dosage?

11 Consider the action of this medication and state why the dosage is so small.

12 Why is Mr Nutzon now receiving continuous monitoring of his blood pressure?

13 The infusion has been in progress for ten minutes. There appears to be no untoward effects from the medication, so the dose is to increase to 1 mcg/kg/minute. What volume/hour should be delivered now?

The dosage rate is increased by 0.5 mcg/kg/minute every ten minutes until a dose of 10 mcg/kg/minute is achieved.

14 a How long would it take for the infusion (from the initial dose) to reach the increase of 10 mcg/kg/minute?

   b What rate of flow will deliver 10 mcg/kg/minute?

Prior to the completion of the infusion containing sodium nitroprusside, verapamil is to be commenced. The order is for 0.24 grams/day, to be given in three equally divided doses. The purpose of this medication for Mr Nutzon is to increase coronary blood flow, which in turn increases oxygen available to the heart.

15 If stock available is 80 mg tablets, how many tablets should be given for a single dose?

16 When you return to duty next morning, one of your tasks is to weigh Mr Nutzon. His current weight is 72.8 kg. Approximately how much fluid has he lost since his admission yesterday?

17 The intravenous digoxin has been reduced to 0.5 mg for today, but it is still to be given BD. Stock is 500 mcg/2 ml. What volume is required for a single dose of this medication?

18 Oral frusemide, 120 mg, is to be given over the next 24 hours, at 06.00 and 12.00. Stock on hand is 40 mg scored tablets. How many tablets/dose should he receive?

19 His intravenous infusion, which commenced at midnight, is to remain in situ and 1 L of 0.9% sodium chloride is to continue dripping at 30 drops/minute. Remembering that a micro-set is in use, calculate the volume/hour he is currently receiving.

20 Today he is permitted 1500 ml of fluid. Taking into account his intravenous infusion, how much oral fluid is he permitted?

EXERCISE FOUR

Mrs Sandy Gray is a 35-year-old primary school teacher who has just been admitted to the ward with Lobar Pneumonia. She admits to feeling unwell for the past two weeks but only sought medical advice when she awoke this morning with chest tightness, a productive cough and fever. She states that she feels very weak and has a 'bad' headache.

Baseline observations include B/P 95/55, pulse 120, weak but regular, temperature 40.2°C and respirations 26, deep and gasping. She states that she has not voided since 16.00 yesterday, and she still feels that she is unable to void urine. Her weight is 55 kg.

Oxygen is commenced at 6 L/minute, an intravenous line is established, a complete blood analysis is carried out, a sputum specimen is collected, a chest X-ray completed and an order for intravenous amoxycillin 1 gram statim is given.

1   1 L of 5% dextrose is to be administered over a 6-hour period. What volume of intravenous fluid should she receive every hour, and if the drop factor for the giving set is 20 drops/ml, how fast should this infusion drip?

Amoxycillin is available as 1 gram of powder in a 10 ml vial for reconstitution. Instructions accompanying the medication indicate that 4.2 ml of sterile water added to the vial will give a concentration of 200 mg/ml.

2   To achieve the above concentration, what volume of fluid has the powder displaced?

Because Amoxycillin is less stable in carbohydrate solutions (eg, dextrose), you are to add the 1 gram of medication to 100 ml of 0.9% sodium chloride via a secondary line, and infuse it over a 30-minute period. The drop factor for this line is also 20 drops/ml.

3   How fast should this infusion drip?

4   If you take into account the two infusions currently being administered, how much intravenous fluid will she receive this hour?

5   Considering her present condition, have you any concerns about giving this volume of fluid over this period of time?

Having settled into the ward, Mrs Gray calls you and asks if you would telephone her husband to bring in her night clothes and several large bottles of Coke as she is very thirsty. She then drifts off to sleep.

Her husband arrives at 11.00 and is very distressed when he is unable to rouse her. The medical officer is notified and, following a discussion with her husband, orders a blood glucose reading immediately. The reading is 54.6 mmol/L. Mrs Gray is transferred to ICU for monitoring and management of Diabetic Ketoacidosis. You seek, and gain permission, to continue assisting in the management of her care.

At 11.30, a Guedel's airway, a urinary catheter, a nasogastric suction catheter, and a central venous line are all inserted, and the dextrose is replaced with 1 L of 0.9% sodium chloride which is to infuse at the rate of 15 ml/minute to increase her circulatory volume.

6 To what speed, in ml/hour, will the infusion pump need to be set to deliver the above order?

The above fluid order, which commenced at 11.30, is to continue until intravascular volume is stabilised as indicated by a normal CVP (Central Venous Pressure) reading and a urinary output of 1 ml/kg of body weight/hour.

7 What CVP reading would be considered normal for Mrs Gray?

8 If her weight is 55 kg, how much urine would indicate to you that stabilisation had occurred when you check the hourly urine measuring container while performing your half hourly checks?

A loading dose of 10 units of intravenous Actrapid is given and then an Actrapid infusion of 0.2 units/kg of body weight/hour is to be set up via a second infusion line. This insulin solution is to have a 1:1 ratio (1 unit of insulin to 1 ml of fluid) and is to be available for 24 hours. The intravenous mode of administration is chosen to ensure absorption because inadequate tissue perfusion is currently present.

9 How much insulin is required for this task?

10 What volume of 0.9% sodium chloride is required for this order?

11 What volume of fluid/hour will deliver the above order?

Following stabilisation of her intravascular volume at 14.00, the 0.9% sodium chloride is removed and replaced with 0.45% sodium chloride, to be infused at the rate of 250 ml/hour. This hypotonic solution is expected to decrease blood osmolarity, as well as decreasing the blood glucose level (BGL) by increasing the urine output.

12 How much fluid was required to stabilise Mrs Gray's intra-vascular volume?

13 Her blood glucose reading is now 37.5. Express the decrease in her BGL as a percentage.

Blood glucose readings are carried out every half hour, and once the reading reaches 15 mmol/L, the infusion of 0.45% sodium chloride is to be replaced with 5% dextrose to prevent hypoglycaemia from developing. The dextrose is commenced at 17.00.

Next morning when you return to duty, Mrs Gray is awake and orientated to time and place. Her CVP reading and her urine output are within acceptable limits and she is taking oral fluids.

14 You check her intravenous infusion and note that it is now dripping at 50 drops/minute. If the drop factor for the giving set is 20 drops/ml, what volume of intravenous fluid is she receiving every hour?

15 She is currently tolerating 100 ml of oral fluid/hour. What is her total hourly volume of fluid?

Her amoxycillin is due and she is to have 0.75 g every six hours. Stock available is 1 gram in a 10 ml vial and the registered nurse asks you to reconstitute this medication to a concentration of 250 mg/ml.

16 If the 1 gram of powder displaces 0.8 ml of fluid, what volume of sterile water is required for this task?

17 What volume should be drawn up for 08.00 dose?

18 You are to add this medication to 50 ml of 0.9% sodium chloride in the burette and infuse it over a 30-minute period. How fast should it drip?

Sliding scale insulin is now to be administered every four hours according to her blood glucose reading. She has been ordered:

Under 7.9 mmol/L.............nil
7.9 to 11.9......................2 units of Actrapid
12 to 15.9........................4 units
16 to 19.9........................6 units
20 to 23.9........................8 units
Above 24 ....notify the medical officer

19 You take her reading and note that it is 12.2. How much insulin should you give her?

She is seen by the medical officer later in the day when her temperature spikes at 41°C. Her fluid intake is increased and she is ordered 240 mg of intravenous gentamicin.

20 a If gentamicin ampoules are available as 80 mg/2 ml, what volume should be drawn up?

b You are to add the gentamicin to 30 ml of fluid into the burette and infuse it over a 20-minute period. How fast should it drip?

EXERCISE FIVE

You have been allocated the care of Mrs Jenny Smith, a 56-year-old woman who was admitted for ongoing treatment of non-Hodgkins Lymphoma. Mrs Smith has a history of Chronic Ischaemic Heart Disease, Hypercholesterolaemia and Hypothyroidism. Mrs Smith has asked you to call her Jenny.

Following the recording of her baseline observations, she is to commence a chemotherapy regime and her first day in hospital is referred to as day –7. You are about to administer her 08.00 medications.

1 Allopurinol 0.3 g, has been ordered. This is a medication to reduce the production of uric acid, a side effect of chemotherapy. If stock available is 300 mg tablets, what should you give her?

2 Because Jenny is prone to viral infections such as Herpes while she is receiving chemotherapy, valaciclovir 500 mg each day has been ordered as a prophylactic measure. If stock available is 0.5 g tablets, what should she be given?

3 For her Hypothyroidism she has been ordered Thyroxine 200 mcg daily. From available stock of 100 mcg tablets, what should you give her?

4 She is currently receiving atorvastatin 20 mg daily to reduce her cholesterol levels. If stock on hand is equivalent to 0.04 g scored tablets, what should she be given?

5 Atenolol 100 mg daily has been ordered to combat Jenny's Hypertension. From available stocks of 50 mg tablets, what should you give her?

6 The antibiotic ciprofloxacin 250 mg has been ordered BD as a prophylactic measure against a broad range of bacteria which could be harmful once Jenny becomes immuno-suppressed. If stock in the ward is 0.5 g scored tablets, what should she be given?

On day –6, a central venous catheter (CVC) is inserted and Jenny is to receive 3 L of intravenous fluid per 24 hours. This CVC will also be used to administer medications such as her chemotherapy and antibiotics.

7 How many ml/hour will Jenny receive from the above order if the drop factor for the giving set is 20 drops/ml, and how fast should the infusion drip?

8 The fact that Jenny has Chronic Ischaemic Heart Disease was taken into account when this fluid order was established and intravenous frusemide 40 mg has been ordered two to 4-hourly PRN, to prevent hypervolaemia. If stock available is 10 mg/ml, what volume needs to be drawn up for this order?

On day –5 Jenny begins her chemotherapy. This medication is given according to the body surface area of the client and is administered by the registered nurse who has been trained to work with cytotoxic therapy. Jenny weighs 55 kg and her height is 160 cm. She is to be weighed twice daily so that fluid accumulation is quickly observed.

9 Using the surface area nomogram provided in the appendix, calculate Jenny's body surface area in m^2.

10 a Etoposide, 200 mg/m^2 of body surface area, is to be added to 1 L of 0.9% sodium chloride and infused over one hour. This drug is a plant alkaloid and it interferes with cell division. How many mg should Jenny receive for this dose?

   b Stock available is 100 mg/5 ml or 500 mg/25 ml. Which will you choose and how much should be drawn up?

   c At 08.00, the first infusion of her chemotherapy is commenced. To what speed will the infusion pump need to be set to deliver the above order in the given time?

Jenny's fluid intake is to continue at the rate of 3 L per day, taking into account the fluid infused while administering the cytotoxic therapy.

11 On completion of the infusion containing etoposide, 0.25 L of 0.9% sodium chloride is commenced, to infuse over a 2-hour period. Calculate the volume per hour that Jenny should receive from this order.

12 Intravenous frusemide, 20 mg is ordered. If stock in the ward is 10 mg/ml, what volume should be given?

On completion of the above infusion at 11.00, Jenny is to receive her next cytotoxic medication. She is to be given cytosine arabinoside (Cytarabine), an anti-neoplastic agent which kills cancer cells. For this medication, she is again to receive 200 mg/m^2 of body surface area BD.

13 a Using the body surface area calculated for the previous medication, what volume should be drawn up from available stock of 100 mg/5 ml?

b The above medication is to be added to 500 ml of 0.9% sodium chloride and infused over one hour. How many ml/hour should the infusion pump be set at to deliver this order?

c On completion of the Cytarabine medicated solution at 12.00, 0.25 L of 0.9% sodium chloride is commenced and is to last for four hours. How many ml/hour will deliver this order?

The Cytarabine order is repeated at 16.00 and this is followed by 0.5 L of 5% dextrose, to infuse overnight, completing at 08.00 next morning.

14 Taking into account the time span for the 0.5 L, what volume per hour should be infused?

Jenny's routine for day –5 was to continue until day –1, which means she was to have five days of this regime. However on day –4 Jenny developed severe nausea and started to vomit. An anti-emetic order was written up for her, allowing her to have 10 mg of metoclopramide three times per day.

15 If metoclopramide is available as 5 mg/ml, what volume should be drawn up for a dose at 09.00?

As Jenny is no longer able to retain oral fluids, the oral ciprofloxacin is discontinued and the medication is now to be administered intravenously. This medication is available in a 100 ml glass bottle with a concentration of 2 mg/ml. It is to be delivered via a secondary line, twice each day, when the chemotherapy is not being infused.

16 **a** How many mg of ciprofloxacin is in the 100 ml bottle?
  b If this medication is to infuse over one hour, with a giving set of 20 drops/ml, how fast should it drip?
  c Remembering that Jenny is now to have an extra 200 ml of medicated solution (due to her antibiotics), how much fluid will need to infuse overnight, and what volume per hour should she receive?

17 At 10.00 Jenny had her weight recorded at 55.6 kg. How much fluid is she currently retaining?

18 Intravenous frusemide, 30 mg is ordered. If stock on hand is 10 mg/ml, what should be drawn up for this order?

Jenny experienced quite a bit of discomfort during the five days of treatment—her white cell count dropped, she lost her hair, and she developed mucositis. On day 0 she completed the cytotoxic regime with the medication melphalan.

19 **a** Melphalan (an anti-neoplastic alkylating agent), 140 mg/m^2 of body surface area, is due to be given via an intravenous push over a 5-minute period. How many mg should Jenny be given?
  b If stock available is 100 mg/10 ml vial, what volume should be drawn up and how should this medication be given over this 5-minute period?

It is day 0 + 2 and Jenny has completed her medication regime. She has received Granocyte (G-CSF) injections for neutropaenia, her allo-purinol tablets have been ceased and her stem cells, collected prior to the cytotoxic therapy, have been infused. Her weight is now 51.7 kg.

20 What percentage of her weight has she lost during the chemo-therapy regime over the past nine days?

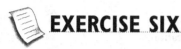

EXERCISE SIX

It is 07.00 and you have just come on duty for the morning shift in the Burns Unit and Mr Ron Kelly, a 60-year-old man, is being admitted to the unit following burns sustained while he was fighting a bushfire earlier this morning. He is displaying signs of shock, has some difficulties breathing and is in severe pain. Oxygen is commenced. He tells you that he weighs 72 kg and is 180 cm tall.

1   Using the nomogram supplied in the index, calculate his body surface area in m².

Assessment of Mr Kelly indicates that he has second degree burns to the front of both legs, his genital area, his abdomen, chest, face and lower right arm.

2   **a** Using the 'Rule of Nines' (see appendix), calculate the percentage of his body that is burned.

      b How much actual body surface area (in m²) is burnt?

An intravenous infusion has been established to assist in replacing his fluid loss. He is to have 2 ml/kg of body weight × the percentage of body burnt, to be given in the first 24 hours. Half of this fluid is to be given in the first eight hours following his burns which occurred at 06.00.

3   **a** Calculate the volume of fluid he should receive in the first 24 hours.

      b What volume is required for the first eight hours?

      c When would you expect the 8-hour fluid order to complete?

4   **a** How many ml/hour will need to be delivered in the first half of this fluid order?

      b How would you expect such a large volume of fluid to be delivered to him?

5   Mr Kelly is to have a statim dose of 15 mg of intravenous morphine to reduce his pain, which must be injected slowly. If stock in the ward is 10 mg/ml, what volume should be drawn up?

Following a Tetanus injection of 250 units of TIG, antibiotics are commenced. He is to have amoxycillin 40 mg/kg of body weight/day, to be given 6-hourly.

6 **a** Calculate his daily dose of this medication.
   b Calculate a single dose of this medication.

Amoxycillin is available as 1 gram of powder in a 10 ml vial. Instructions accompanying this medication indicate that the powder will displace 0.7 ml of fluid on reconstitution.

7 **a** How much sterile water is required to reconstitute this medication to a solution with a concentration of 200 mg/ml?
   b What volume of medication should be drawn up for his first dose?

8 This medication is to be added to a 50 ml bag of 0.9% sodium chloride via a secondary line with a drop factor of 20 drops/ml and infused over a 15-minute period. How fast will the infusion need to drip to fulfil this order?

It is 10.30 and you are assisting the registered nurse to set up a morphine infusion to control Mr Kelly's ongoing pain. This infusion solution is to contain 60 mg of morphine. The total volume required for this medication infusion is 60 ml.

9 **a** If stock available is 10 mg/ml, how many ml of morphine is required for this task?
   b Remembering that the total volume for this infusion is 60 ml, how much fluid is required to complete this task?

10 **a** Mr Kelly is to commence this infusion with a 4 mg/hour dose of morphine. How many ml/hour will deliver this order?
   b What is the concentration, in mg/ml, of this medicated solution?
   c How long would you expect this medicated infusion to last?

At 11.30 Mr Kelly becomes quite nauseated and begins to dry retch. A nasogastric, low suction tube is introduced and intravenous metoclopramide hydrochloride (Maxolon) 7.5 mg is ordered.

11 If ward stock available is 10 mg/2 ml, what volume of Maxolon should be drawn up?

When you return from lunch at 13.50, the registered nurse is preparing Mr Kellys fifth bag of infusion solution, which is a bag of Ringer's Lactate solution.

12 a How much fluid will Mr Kelly have in the next sixteen hours?
  b To what rate of flow will the volumetric infusion pump need to be adjusted?
  c State the purpose of the Ringer's Lactate solution with regards to Mr Kelly's present condition.

Next morning when you return to duty, you are to continue working with the same registered nurse to care for Mr Kelly. Today's fluid intake is to begin with 2000 ml of 5% dextrose in water and is to be infused at the rate of 250 ml per hour for the next 24 hours.

13 How much fluid will be charted on his fluid balance chart in relation to this order for day two?

Following a very limited morning wash, Mr Kelly says that his pain is unbearable. The medical officer orders a bolus dose of 8 mg of morphine over a 4-minute period.

14 a Remembering that this infusion is still the one you assisted in setting up yesterday, how many mg/minute will need to be delivered?
  b How many ml of solution will deliver the calculated mg/minute?

15 To what speed will you need to adjust the infusion pump to deliver the ordered dose in the specified time?

Mr Kelly's morphine infusion completes at 09.30, and he is to transfer to a Patient Controlled Analgesia (PCA), via an intravenous line. At 10.30 you are observing the two registered nurses who are setting up this line. Mr Kelly is to have 60 mg of morphine in a 60 ml solution of sterile sodium chloride. This is to be delivered via a syringe pump connected to an intravenous cannula in his arm.

16 a If the morphine available in the unit is 10 mg/ml, how much sterile sodium chloride is required for this task?
  b Mr Kelly is not to be given a 'loading dose of morphine'. Why would this be so?
  c A bolus dose of 1 mg of morphine is available for Mr Kelly's use and there is a lock-out period of five minutes. What does this mean?

17 The registered nurse asks you to explain to her what instructions should be given to Mr Kelly regarding the use of his PCA. What information would you give her?

18 **a** What observations should be made of Mr Kelly while his PCA is in progress?

b What information (with regards to the PCA) should be given to his relatives when they come to visit?

A routine observation of Mr Kelly's intravenous site indicates that the fluid is no longer infusing into the vein but is 'running into the tissues'.

19 **a** What objective data would suggest that the swelling at the infusion site was not thrombophlebitis?

b What is the medical term for fluid leaking into the tissues?

20 A decision is made to insert a CVC when the peripheral line is removed. State why this line is preferable to other peripheral lines.

EXERCISE SEVEN

Mrs Robyn Murray is a 30-year-old woman who has just been transferred to the ward following surgery to clip a ruptured subarachnoid artery and to evacuate an intracranial haematoma. On transfer to the ward she is conscious but almost immediately has a 30-second tonic–clonic seizure.

1 A central venous infusion of nimodipime (a medication that prevents cerebral arterial spasm) is in progress. Mrs Murray is having 30 mcg/kg/hour. If her weight is 67 kg, how many mg of this medication is she to receive each hour?

2 The above infusion of nimodipine is available as 10 mg in a 50 ml bottle, and is delivered via a volumetric pump on a secondary line. What volume should be delivered per hour?

Nimodopine should always be delivered via a CVC using a 3-way stopcock and polyethylene tubing because polyvinylchloride tubing absorbs nimodopine. It should also be infused concurrently with compatible intravenous solutions such as 0.9% sodium chloride or 5% dextrose at a 1:4 ratio.

3 5% dextrose is currently infusing. Taking into account the above information, what volume of this fluid would you expect to see infusing each hour?

4 Mrs Murray states that she has a headache and would like pain relief. She is permitted subcutaneous morphine 5 mg, two- to four-hourly PRN. Her last dose was at 08.15 and it is now 10.20. Is she permitted another dose at this time?

5 If so, the stock of morphine available is 10 mg/ml, so what volume should be drawn up?

6 If the normal dosage range of subcutaneous morphine is 5–20 mg 4/24 PRN, is her ordered dose within these limits?

7 At 10.40 Mrs Murray calls you and says she feels nauseous. Checking her notes you see that intravenous metoclopramide 10 mg may be given 6/24 PRN. If stock on hand is 10 mg/2 ml, what volume should be given?

8 According to the MIMS Annual (2001) metoclopramide dosages should not exceed 30 mg/day, especially if the client has suffered a head injury, because this drug has the potential to mask symptoms such as cerebral irritation. Why might Mrs Murray be given more than the recommended dose in this instance?

9 Mrs Murray has a past history of Crohn's Disease, so she is to continue her usual dose of prednisolone to reduce the immune response. Because nausea is a problem, she is currently to have 40 mg/day, to be given BD via the subcutaneous route. If stock is 40 mg/ml, what volume should she be given?

10 Another medication for Crohn's Disease is the immuno-suppressant drug azathioprine. This medication is available as 50 mg of powder for reconstitution with 5 ml of sterile water. Mrs Murray is to have 50 mg daily. Because the medication is a very irritating solution, it is to added to 50 ml bag of 0.9% sodium chloride and infused over a 30-minute period. How fast should this order drip?

11 Intravenous phenytoin (Dilantin) 0.4 grams per day is to be given to BD to limit seizure activities by reducing hyperexcitability

especially in the motor cortex. If stock available is 100 mg/2 ml, what volume should be drawn up for a single dose?

It is day four post surgery and Mrs Murray's condition improves each day. Her nausea and headaches have decreased significantly. She is now taking and tolerating a light diet, but a peripheral infusion continues, mainly to keep the line open in case of an emergency. She is having 1 L over 24 hours. Her medications are now being given orally.

12 On checking her infusion you note that the 0.9% sodium chloride is dripping at 14 drops/minute. Is this the correct rate of flow for the given order?

13 Metoclopramide continues to be given and she is to have 5 mg TDS. If stock is 10 mg scored tablets, what should she receive?

14 Nimodipine 60 mg is to be given 4/24. If stock available is 30 mg tablets, how many tablets/dose should she be given?

15 Following her first shower after surgery, Mrs Murray asks for pain relief. She is now permitted Oxycodone 7.5 mg 4/24 PRN. If tablets available are 5 mg, what should you give her?

16 Her 0.4 g of phenytoin is to be given QID. If stock available is 100 mg capsules, how many capsules should she receive per dose?

17 The prednisolone is reduced to 30 mg/day, to be given TDS. If stock is 5 mg tablets, how many tablets should she receive per dose?

18 Azathioprine 50 mg is to be given BD. If stock is 50 mg tablets, what should you give her for a single dose?

19 On day five Mrs Murray's infusion is to be removed on completion. She asks you how long the remaining 70 ml will last as she would like to walk to the kiosk. If it is dripping at 14 drops/minute, what do you tell her?

20 It is day seven and Mrs Murray's sutures have just been removed from her scalp. She says it is rather sore there now and asks for some pain relief. Paracetamol 1 g is ordered. How many tablets should she be given if stock is 500 mg/tablet?

EXERCISE EIGHT

It is your final clinical placement as an undergraduate student and you have chosen to work in the Emergency Department of a large metropolitan hospital.

At 07.30 a 19-year-old woman, Lisa Brown, is brought to the Emergency Department by ambulance from the airport, following a flight from London. On admission she is extremely anxious, has chest pain, dyspnoea, diaphoresis and haemoptysis. She tells you that her lower right leg is very painful.

Oxygen is commenced, oxygen saturation levels are monitored, and an intravenous line is established. Immediate laboratory studies include ABG, ECG and chest radiography. Lisa is to be transferred to ICU as soon as a bed becomes available. Meanwhile, a provisional diagnosis of Pulmonary Embolus following a Deep Vein Thrombosis (DVT) is made.

1 1 L of 0.9% sodium chloride is to infuse over twelve hours. What volume of fluid will be put into the burette each hour, and how many drops/minute will deliver this order if the drop factor is 20 drops/ml?

2 Intravenous morphine 8 mg is ordered to reduce her pain and anxiety. It also assists by decreasing preload and afterload (circulatory depression is one of the adverse effects of morphine), thus limiting pulmonary hypertension and ventricular strain. If stock is 10 mg/ml, what volume is required?

3 The morphine is to be delivered over a 4-minute period. How should this be achieved?

Intravenous Actilyse 100 mg has been ordered. This medication (recombinant tissue plasminogen activator) acts to convert plasminogens to the enzyme fibrinogen, thus dissolving fibrin clots. Lisa is to have a loading dose of 15 mg, followed by 50 mg over the next 30 minutes, with the remaining 35 mg to be delivered over the next hour.

4 If stock available is 50 mg/50 ml, what volume should be drawn up and given for the initial bolus dose?

5 a The 50 mg dose is to be infused over a 30-minute period, using a volumetric pump. To what speed, in ml/hour, should the pump be set?

   b What volume/hour will deliver the remaining 35 mg?

Following laboratory reports on completion of the thrombolytic therapy, anticoagulant therapy is commenced. Lisa is to have a bolus dose of Heparin, 80 units/kg of body weight. Lisa weighs 60 kg. This is to be followed by 1000 units of Heparin/hour for 24 hours.

6 Calculate the bolus dose of Heparin, and state the volume required if stock on hand is 5000 units/ml. What type of syringe should be used to measure this intravenous medication?

7 25 000 units (1 ml) of Heparin is to be added in a 100 ml bag of 0.9% sodium chloride and delivered via a volumetric pump. How many ml/hour will deliver the ordered dose of 1000 units/hour?

Lisa is transferred to ICU at 10.30, just as another ambulance arrives with a 32-year-old man with a severe head injury. Colin Bright stepped backwards from the tray of a truck while unloading goods and fell, hitting his head on the concrete roadside curb.

On admission he had a large head wound, was losing a lot of blood, but was alert and orientated. An MRI scan is ordered, followed by the suturing of his head wound in the Emergency theatre. While waiting for the ordered investigations to be carried out, he has a seizure and lapses into unconsciousness. A statim dose of Osmitrol 20% is ordered to be delivered over a 30-minute period at the rate of 200 mg/kg of body weight. An indwelling urinary catheter is inserted.

8 a How many grams should be given for the initial dose if his weight is 75 kg?

   b What is the concentration (in mg/ml) of the 500 ml of Osmitrol 20% solution?

9 What volume of fluid contains the ordered dose of 200 mg/kg?

10 This medication is to be delivered via a volumetric pump. To what speed (in ml/hr) will the pump need to be set to deliver this large volume of medication in the ordered 30 minutes?

11 Osmitrol is a powerful osmotic diuretic which has the potential to

reduce intracranial pressure by creating an osmotic gradient between plasma and CSF (cerebrospinal fluid). What minimum volume of urine/hour would be acceptable for this client?

12 a On completion of the initial bolus dose, the infusion of Osmitrol is to progress at 1.5 g/kg/day. Using a 20% solution in 0.5 L, calculate the mg/hour required.

b Calculate the volume/hour that will deliver the above dose.

Mr Bright is transferred to the MRI department and you are asked to assist with the management of Mr Jack Frost, a 50-year-old male who is admitted with a severe Asthma attack. On admission his breathing is laboured and wheezy, with the use of accessory muscles being visible. Cyanosis is present. He is nursed in an upright position, oxygen is commenced, and an intravenous infusion is established. He is ordered pulmonary function studies, arterial blood gases, and the following medications.

13 Following an inhalation of salbutamol (a bronchodilator) which had a minimal effect, he is ordered intravenous salbutamol 300 mcg, to be given over one minute. If stock is 0.5 mg/ml, what volume should be given?

14 His intravenous order is for 4 L over a 24-hour period. Calculate the volume of fluid/hour, and the number of drops/minute that will deliver this order if the drop factor is 20 drops/ml.

15 Intravenous aminophylline 5 mg/kg of body weight is ordered as a loading dose, which will increase bronchial smooth muscle relaxation. Mr Frost weighs 75 kg and stock available is 250 mg/ 10 ml. Calculate the volume required.

16 The loading dose is to be added to the 85 ml in the burette and infused over a 30-minute period. How fast should it drip?

17 Explain why intravenous aminophylline needs to be introduced slowly when given as a bolus dose.

18 On completion of the bolus dose, he is ordered a continuous aminophylline infusion at the rate of 0.5 mg/kg/hour for the next twelve hours. Calculate the volume of aminophylline required for this order.

19 The aminophylline is to be added to a 250 ml bag of 0.9% sodium chloride and infused via a secondary line through a volumetric pump. Calculate the rate of flow in ml/hour for this order.

20 Mr Frost is commenced on 60 mg of prednisolone per day, for the first 24 hours, to be given QID. If stock on hand is 30 mg tablets, what should he be given for a single dose?

EXERCISE NINE

Ms Vanessa Cox is a 20-year-old woman who has been brought into the Emergency Department by the Retrieval Team after being trapped in a motor vehicle for 90 minutes, following an accident where she was a passenger in a car which hit a light pole at considerable speed.

On admission at 06.30, she was irritable and most uncooperative. Oxygen was continued and a CVC & IDC (indwelling urinary catheter) inserted. 0.5 L of 4% dextrose in 0.18% sodium chloride was commenced via a volumetric pump. An intracranial pressure monitor was inserted which revealed a raised intracranial pressure.

An immediate CT scan highlighted her numerous injuries. She sustained multiple contusions of the head, a fractured base of the skull, numerous facial fractures, a comminuted fracture of both the left ulna and femur and a compound, comminuted fracture of her right tibia and fibula. There was evidence of significant blood loss.

1 How long would you expect this bag of fluid to last if 80 ml/hour was to be delivered?

Pain relief was the next priority for Vanessa. At 07.30 an intravenous infusion of morphine 60 mg and midazolam 30 mg was organised. The two medications were to be delivered via a syringe driver connected to an intravenous cannula in her right arm. The total volume of this solution is 60 ml and is expected to last approximately 20 hours. You are assisting two registered nurses set up this infusion.

2 What volume of morphine is required for this task, if stock available is 15 mg/ml?

3 If midazolam is available as 15 mg/3 ml, what volume is required for this order?

4 How much 0.9% sodium chloride is required to make up a volume of 60 ml?

5 This infusion is to begin with a bolus dose of 2 ml of this medicated solution. How many mg of each drug will the 2 ml deliver?

6 **a** What is the concentration of both the morphine and the midazolam, in mg/ml, of this solution?

   b At what speed, in ml/hour, should this infusion be maintained to deliver the prescribed dose in the ordered time?

7 State the purpose of combining the midazolam with the morphine, and explain how this is expected to enhance Vanessa's comfort.

At 08.00, 500 ml of intravenous succinylated gelatin (Gelofusine) is to be given. This solution is a colloidal plasma volume substitute, which is to be delivered via the infusion pump, and you have been asked to warm it to 37°C. You are aware that reactions to this solution sometimes occur.

8 You have been asked to commence this infusion at the rate of 25 ml/hour for the first fifteen minutes. Why would this be so?

9 The remainder of the solution is to complete in 45 minutes. To what speed, in ml/hour, should the infusion pump be set to fulfil this order?

10 State the purpose of administering this solution to Vanessa, and why were you asked to warm it?

Vanessa is transferred to ICU at 09.00 and is resting quietly. You have sought and gained permission to assist with her subsequent care. Surgery to her injuries has been postponed for the time being. An antibiotic regime is commenced to help protect her from infection. This regime is commenced with a 400 mg dose of intravenous gentamicin.

11 **a** From available stock of 80 mg/2 ml, what volume of gentamicin should be drawn up and given?

   b According to MIMS (2001), the usual dose of gentamicin is 80 mg TDS. Why do you think that such a large dose of this medication is being administered to Vanessa?

Intravenous cefoxitin sodium, 1 gram TDS, is also commenced. This medication is available as 1 gram of powder in a 10 ml vial for reconstitution. Instructions accompanying the medication indicate that the powder will displace 0.8 ml of fluid when a solution is formed.

12 What volume of sterile water is required to reconstitute the above medication to a concentration of 250 mg/ml?

13 This medication is to be added to a 50 ml bag of 0.9% sodium chloride and infused over 30 minutes. If the drop factor for this line is 20 drops/ml, how fast should this solution drip?

At 09.50, Vanessa (weighing 50 kg) becomes restless and, within a few minutes, has a seizure. Intravenous phenytoin, 100 mcg/kg/minute is ordered. 300 mg of phenytoin is to be added to a 50 ml bag of 0.9% sodium chloride and infused at room temperature to prevent precipitation.

14 If phenytoin is available as 100 mg/2 ml, what volume should be added to the bag of 0.9% sodium chloride?

15 This medicated solution is to infuse over a 10-minute period and the drop factor for this line is 15 drops/ml. How fast should the line drip?

At 12.15 a decision is made to transfer Vanessa to the Emergency operating suite to stabilise her fractures. The fractured bones in her limbs are immobilised by pins and/or plates. A nasogastric tube is inserted and Vanessa is returned to ICU at 15.30.

16 Flagyl 0.5 grams is to be given BD via the nasogastric tube. If stock available is 200 mg/5 ml, calculate the volume to be poured and given.

As a result of the facial damage and extreme stress that Vanessa sustained in the accident, a medication to inhibit the production of hydrochloric acid has been ordered. Intravenous pantoprazole, 40 mg/day, is to be given. Stock available is 40 mg of powder in a 10 ml vial for reconstitution.

17 Following reconstitution of this medication with 10 ml of 0.9% sodium chloride, it is added to a 50 ml bag of 5% dextrose and is to infuse over ten minutes using the 15 drops/ml giving set. Calculate the rate of flow, in drops/minute, for this infusion.

18 State the reason why this medication is considered important for Vanessa's recovery.

At 16.30 Vanessa is awake and showing signs of distress. She is to receive a bolus dose of 3 mg of her pain medication, morphine and midazolam, over three minutes.

19 a How many mg of morphine/minute should she receive from this order?

b Referring back to Q 6a for the concentration of this solution, calculate the volume of fluid/minute that is required to deliver the ordered dose?

20 To what speed, in ml/hour, should the syringe driver be adjusted to deliver the ordered dose within the prescribed time?

EXERCISE TEN

You are continuing with your care of Vanessa Cox in ICU and it is day two following her motor vehicle accident (MVA). Her intracranial pressure remains higher than normal, she is febrile and has a productive cough.

Her pain control medication of 60 mg morphine and 30 mg midazolam in 60 ml is continuing at 2 ml/hour with the desired effect. Following handover you visit Vanessa. She does not respond to your voice nor does she appear to understand that you are talking to her, but she is moving her right arm. At 08.00, she is seen by the neurologist who orders the following changes to her regime. She is to have:

- Intravenous erythromycin 100 mg BD
- Intravenous ticarcillin 3 grams TDS
- Intravenous gentamicin 320 mg today
- Oral Flagyl 0.75 grams TDS via the nasogastric tube
- A statim dose of 25 grams of Mannitol, to be delivered at the rate of 200 mg/kg/hour, and Vanessa weighs 50 kg.

1 Mantol is available as 10% in 1000 ml, or 10% in 500 ml, or 20% in 1000 ml or 20% in 500 ml. Which bag of stock solution would you choose to use for the total dose of 25 grams?

2 State the reason why the Mannitol has been ordered for Vanessa.

3 What volume of fluid is required from your chosen bag for the above order?

4 **a** This infusion is to be delivered via an infusion pump at the rate of 200 mg/kg/hour, until 25 grams has been administered. How many ml/hour will fulfil this order?
   b How long will it take to deliver the 25 grams of Mannitol?

5 Stock of erythromycin is a 10 ml vial containing 300 mg of powder. This medication is to be reconstituted with 6 ml of sterile water to form a concentration of approximately 50 mg/ml. What volume should be drawn up for her first dose?

6 **a** This medication is to be further diluted with 0.9% sodium chloride to a concentration of 1 mg/ml. Which will you choose for this task: a 50 ml or a 100 ml bag of normal saline?
   b Using the 15 drops/ml infusion set, how fast should this medication drip to complete in 20 minutes?

7 The antibiotic ticarcillin sodium is due now. She is to have 3 grams 6-hourly. If the maximum dose of this medication for a person of Vanessa's size is 300 mg/kg/day, is this dose within acceptable limits?

8 Vanessa's gentamicin is also due. She is to have 320 mg today. From available stock of 80 mg/2 ml, what volume is required?

9 **a** What volume of Flagyl is required from the available stock of 200 mg/5 ml?
   b Prior to administering the above medication, you are to mix it at a 1 to 1 ratio with tap water. What volume of fluid would you then introduce into nasogastric tube?

As part of your ongoing management of Vanessa, you are to record her urinary output every 30 minutes. From 07.00 to 09.30, Vanessa's urinary output was 150 ml. It is now 10.00 and 146 ml of urine has dripped into the bag since it was last emptied at 09.30.

10 Would you have any concerns about this increase in her urine output, and if so, what would you do with this information?

From 10.00 to 10.30, the urine output for Vanessa was 152 ml. She is seen by the neurologist and ordered 10 mcg of intravenous desmopressin acetate (Minirin) statim. This medication is given to reduce the effects of a damaged pituitary gland (as a consequence of her head injuries), which has resulted in a reduction in the production of ADH (Antidiuretic Hormone).

11 a Minirin is available as 40 mcg/ml. What volume is needed for the above order?

   b What type of syringe would be the most accurate for this medication administration?

At 12.00, a blood glucose measurement is ordered, and the reading is 8.2 mm/L. An Actrapid infusion is to be established at the rate of 0.2 units/kg/hour. This infusion is to have a total of 50 ml of fluid, with a concentration of 1 unit of insulin per ml of fluid.

12 How many units of insulin are required for this task, and how many ml would contain the ordered dose?

13 This medication is to be delivered via the infusion pump. How many ml/hour is required for this order?

Your supervising registered nurse asks you to flush Vanessa's CVC line with a Heparin solution, 500 units in 10 ml of 0.9% sodium chloride. Heparin is available as 5000 units in one ml.

14 a What volume of Heparin is required for this order, and what type of syringe would be most suitable to use?

   b 0.9% sodium chloride is available in a 10 ml ampoule. How will you prepare this solution for the task in hand?

At 13.00 Vanessa is having difficulty in breathing. A decision is made to ventilate her and transfer her to the operating theatre for a bifrontal decompressive craniotomy and elevation of depressed facial fractures. On her return to ICU at 15.00, she has a tracheostomy tube in place, connected to the ventilator. She is not responding to any stimuli, so her medications for pain relief are temporarily suspended. Two units of packed cells (0.4 L each) have been ordered, to be given as soon as they arrive in the department. Her 5% dextrose solution is removed and replaced by 100 ml of 0.9% sodium chloride.

15 a The 100 ml of 0.9% sodium chloride is to infuse via a macro-dropper. How many drops/minute will deliver 2 ml/minute?

   b How long would you expect the 100 ml infusion to take to complete?

16 Why were you asked to replace the dextrose infusion with 100 ml of normal saline?

The blood arrives in the ward as the 0.9% sodium chloride infusion completes. Following the checking procedure that is carried out by you and your supervising registered nurse, the blood is commenced.

17 You are to commence each unit of blood at fifteen drops/minute for 15 minutes. Why is this so?

18 The remainder of the blood is to be delivered at the rate of 40 drops/minute. How long will each unit take to complete?

At 16.00 Vanessa has another seizure. Intravenous phenytoin 150 mg is to given over a 5-minute period. Stock is 100 mg/2 ml.

19 a What volume of phenytoin is required for the above order?

   b How many mg/minute should be infused for this order?

   c What volume of fluid will contain the dose/minute?

At 16.20, a blood glucose measurement shows a reading of 7.2 mm/L. An order is given to reduce the rate of flow of the Actrapid infusion to 5 ml/hour.

20 How many units of insulin per hour would Vanessa receive from this action?

Vanessa made a slow recovery, leaving ICU after 3½ weeks. She regained her strength, skills and confidence over the next three months in a rehabilitation unit.

 # ANSWERS

EXERCISE ONE

   1 2 tablets

   2 a 2 tablets/hour   **b** 8 grams

3 **a** 67 drops/minute, at 19.00
  b Potassium   **c** Abdominal cramps, weakness, fatigue

4 **a** 65% survival rate
  b If 70% = 350, then 1% = 5. Therefore 30% = 150 making a total, 350 + 150 = 500

5 15 ml

6 Intake 5000 ml, output 4700 ml. The fluid has probably been absorbed by the large bowel.

7 **a** To reduce anxiety and to dry up secretions of the mouth
  b 1.4 ml   **c** 1 ml

8 250 ml/hour and 83 drops/minute

9 120 ml/hour

10 30 ml/hour or 0.5 ml/kg of body weight/hour

11 **a** 3 mg/ml   **b** 5 ml/hour   **c** 15 mg/hour
  d Yes, a maximum dose at 50 mg/3 hours = 400 mg/day
  e Check that her respiratory rate is within normal limits and that her oxygen 'sats' are satisfactory.

12 **a** 0.4 ml of fluid   **b** 3.3 ml   **c** 47 drops/minute

13 **a** 0.8 ml   **b** Give 0.2 ml/minute

14 **a** 3 mg/minute   **b** 1 ml   **c** 60 ml/hour
  d Ensure that the rate of flow is returned to the ordered dose and check that her respirations and pain levels are satisfactory.

15 **a** 150 ml/hour   **b** 33 drops/minute
  c At 14.30 (will take 7 hours to complete)

16 **a** 600 ml intake
  b To prevent haemolysis—dextrose causes red blood cell aggregation
  c 67 drops/minute

17 **a** 15 drops/minute
  b The reaction, should one occur, is reduced with a slower rate of flow and observed earlier.

  c 33 drops/minute

18 **a** 60 ml/hour   **b** At 09.45

19 $1\frac{1}{2}$ tablets

20 .Constipation is common. Encourage high-fibre foods and extra fluids.

EXERCISE TWO

1 900 mcg or 0.9 mg

2 **a** 14 mg   **b** 0.93 ml   **c** A 1 ml insulin syringe

3 **a** 75 ml/hour   **b** 13 hours 20 minutes
  c He would need constant observation.

4 1 tablet/dose

5 a 8.75 mg/dose and 1.75 ml/dose

6 8 ml

7 5 ml

8 1 ml

9 **a** 60 ml/hour   **b** 160 mg/hour   **c** 30 ml/hour

10 **a** 1.6 ml
  b If infused too fast, hypotension and syncope could result.
  c It can be given with either 5% or 10% dextrose or 0.9% sodium chloride in a 250 ml solution. This amount of extra fluid would be undesirable for this man. It should not be mixed with any other medication.

11 0.25 ml or 25 units in a 0.5 ml insulin syringe

12 15 ml

13 **a** 52.5 mg   **b** 105 ml/hour

14 **a** 35 mg   **b** 35 ml/hour

15 **a** 45 ml/hour   **b** 22 hours 13 minutes
  c At 02.13 tomorrow

16 a 10 ml/hour **b** 160 units/ml **c** 25 hours
d 55 ml/hour

17 0.5 ml

18 1.5 ml

19 a 3 mg/dose **b** $1\frac{1}{2}$ tablets

20 a Aspirin should be avoided while taking warfarin because it could potentiate the action of the warfarin.
b Report the information to the registered nurse supervising your care.

EXERCISE THREE

1 3.2 kg

2 3200 ml or 3.2 L

3 8 ml

4 1.5 ml

5 2 ml

6 a 40 ml, to deliver a more accurate and slower dose
b 12.5 hours

7 50 mg

8 It will decrease the circulatory overload by allowing more blood to reach the peripheral circulation.

9 Because Nitroprusside decomposes when exposed to light

10 22.5 ml/hour

11 It has the potential to cause excessive hypotension in larger doses, and it could also have a profound diuretic effect because it is being given with a diuretic.

12 Sodium nitroprusside is a potent, rapidly acting venous and arterial vasodilator and has the potential to cause severe hypotension.

13 45 ml/hour

14 **a** 3 hours 10 minutes   **b** 450 ml/hour

15 1 tablet/dose

16 2200 ml or 2.2 L

17 1 ml/dose

18 $1\frac{1}{2}$ tablets

19 30 ml/hour

20 780 ml

EXERCISE FOUR

1   167 ml/hour, 56 drops/minute

2   0.8 ml

3   70 drops/minute

4   272 ml (167 + 100 + 5)

5   No, she is extremely dehydrated

6   900 ml/hour

7   3–5 mm

8   28–30 ml per 30-minute period

9   264 units

10 264 ml

11 11 ml/hour

12 2250 ml

13 Approximately 31%

14 150 ml

15 250 ml

16 3.2 ml of sterile water

17 3 ml

18 35 drops/minute

19 4 units

20 **a** 6 ml   **b** 36 drops/minute

EXERCISE FIVE

1 1 tablet

2 1 tablet

3 2 tablets

4 1/2 tablet

5 2 tablets

6 1/2 tablet

7 **a** 125 ml/hour   **b** 42 drops/minute

8 4 ml

9 1.55 m^2

10 **a** 310 mg/dose   **b** 500 mg/25 ml, volume 15.5 ml
    c 1000 ml/hour

11 125 ml/hour

12 2 ml

13 **a** 15.5 ml   **b** 515 ml/hour   **c** 62.5 ml/hour

14 33.3 ml/hour

15 2 ml/dose

16 **a** 200 mg   **b** 33 drops/minute
    c 300 ml/night, 20 ml/hour

17 600 ml is being retained

18 3 ml

19 **a** 217 mg   **b** 21.7ml; 4.34 ml/min

20 6% weight loss

EXERCISE SIX

1 1.9 m^2

2 a 46% **b** 0.87 m^2

3 a 6624 ml **b** 3312 ml **c** At 14.00

4 a 473 ml/hour **b** Via a CVC and a volumetric pump

5 1.5 ml

6 a 2880 mg **b** 720 mg

7 a 4.3 ml of sterile water **b** 3.6 ml

8 72 drops/minute

9 a 6 ml **b** 54 ml

10 a 4 ml/hr **b** 1mg/ml **c** 15 hours

11 1.5 ml

12 a 3312 ml **b** 207 ml/hr
   c to maintain his electrolyte balance

13 6 L

14 a 2 mg/minute **b** 2 ml

15 120 ml/hour for 4 minutes

16 a 54 ml
   b He has been on continuous morphine.
   c He can only have 1 mg every five minutes, no matter how often he presses the button for a dose.

17 He should push the button when he feels that his pain is increasing in severity, before it gets really bad, and he should let the staff know if he feels that his pain is not being relieved.

18 a His respirations and oxygen saturation levels need constant monitoring for signs of respiratory depression.
   b His relatives should not try to push the pain control button for him; Mr Kelly is the only person who should.

19 a If fluid is escaping into the surrounding tissues, the area will be swollen, cool and pale rather than warm and pink as with phlebitis.

    b Extravasation

20 Fluids can be given via this route with minimal effects to the blood vessels, and greater volumes can be given if necessary.

EXERCISE SEVEN

1 2.01 mg/hour

2 10 ml/hour

3 40 ml/hour

4 Yes, two hours have pased since her last dose

5 0.5 ml

6 Yes, her maximum dose order is 60 mg/24 hours

7 2 ml/dose

8 It is important that she avoids vomiting as this has the potential to raise the ICP (intracranial pressure).

9 0.5 ml/dose

10 37 drops/minute

11 4 ml/dose

12 Yes, 14 drops/minute is the correct rate of flow

13 1/2 tablet/dose

14 2 tablets/dose

15 $1\frac{1}{2}$ tablets

16 1 capsule/dose

17 2 tablets/dose

18 1 tablet/dose

19 It will last 1 hour and 40 minutes

20 2 tablets

EXERCISE EIGHT

1 83 ml/hour and 28 drops/minute

2 0.8 ml

3 Give 2 mg/minute

4 15 ml

5 **a** 100 ml/hour   **b** 35 ml/hour

6 4800 units, 0.96 ml or 96 units using a one ml insulin syringe

7 4 ml/hour

8 **a** 15 grams   **b** 200 mg/ml

9 200 mg × 75 kg × 150 ml ÷ 100 000 = 75 ml/hour

10 150 ml/hour

11 1 ml/kg of body weight/hour or up to 60 ml/hour

12 **a** 4687.5 mg/hour or 112 500 mg ÷ 24 hours
    b 23.43 ml/hour

13 0.6 ml

14 167 ml/hour and 56 drops/minute

15 15 ml

16 67 drops/minute

17 Because it can cause hypotension due to its CNS and cardio-vascular stimulating effects if given too fast.

18 18 ml

19 22.33 ml/hour

20 1/2 tablet/dose

EXERCISE NINE

1 6.25 hours or 6 hours 15 minutes

2 4 ml

3 6 ml

4 50 ml

5 2 mg of morphine and 1 mg of midazolam

6 **a** Morphine 1 mg/ml, midazolam 0.5 mg/ml
   b 3 ml/hour

7 Midazolam acts as a sedative, and when combined with morphine, it reduces anxiety and pain (MIMS, 2001, 3–251).

8 For early detection of a reaction, with minimal harm to the client.

9 658 ml/hour   (493.75 ÷ 45 × 60)

10 Purpose: to replenish circulatory volume. Cold fluid could induce or enhance shock when delivered at such a fast speed.

11 **a** 10 ml
    b She has a very high potential for the development of infection, in particular, the head wounds.

12 3.2 ml

13 36 drops/minute

14 6 ml

15 84 drops/minute

16 12.5 ml

17 90 drops/minute

18 Vanessa has the potential to develop a stress ulcer in the GI tract, hence a reduction in the hydrochloric acid will minimise harm.

19 **a** 1 mg of morphine/minute   **b** 1 ml/minute

20 60 ml/hour for 3 minutes

EXERCISE TEN

1 The 10% in 500 ml bag would be the closest to what is required.

2 Mannitol is a diuretic. By reducing brain mass (its diuretic action) there is a reduction in intracranial pressure.

3 250 ml

4 **a** 100 ml/hour   **b** 2 hours 30 minutes

5 2 ml

6 **a** 100 ml bag   **b** 76–77 drops/minute

7 Yes, she will have 12 grams/day and is permitted up to 15 grams per day.

8 8 ml

9 **a** 18.75 ml/dose   **b** 37.5 ml

10 Yes. However it could be the diuretic effect of the Mannitol. Report to the person in charge.

11 **a** 0.25 ml   **b** A 0.5 ml insulin syringe

12 50 units and 0.5 ml

13 10 ml/hour

14 **a** 0.1 ml and use a 0.5 ml insulin syringe
    b Draw up the Heparin in an insulin syringe and put it aside. Open a 10 ml vial of normal saline and add the Heparin. Use a 10 ml syringe to mix and draw up.

15 **a** 40 drops/minute   **b** 50 minutes

16 Dextrose has the potential to cause aggregation of the red blood cells.

17 For early detection of a reaction with minimal exposure to the client of the agents causing the reaction.

18 3 hours 14 minutes

19 **a** 3 ml   **b** 30 mg/minute   **c** 0.6 ml

20 5 units/hour

APPENDIX 1.1

Nomogram for an adult

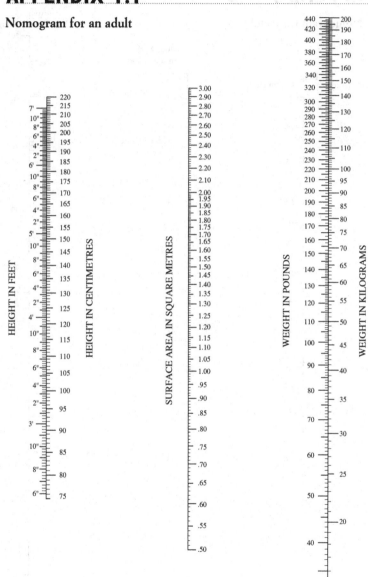

Source: Boothby and Sandiford (1921)

APPENDIX 1.2

Nomogram for a child

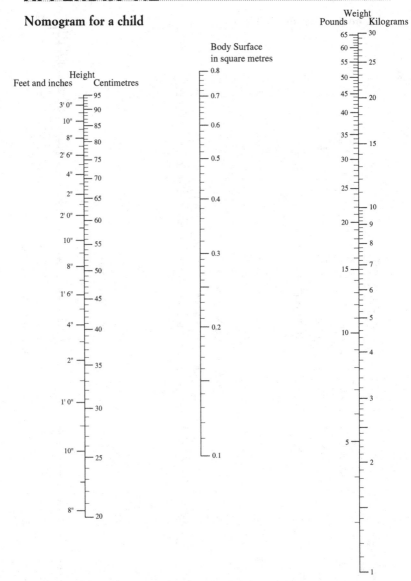

Weight
Pounds · Kilograms

Body Surface
in square metres

Height
Feet and inches · Centimetres

Source: Du Bois (1936)

APPENDIX 2.1

The 'Rule of Nines' for an adult

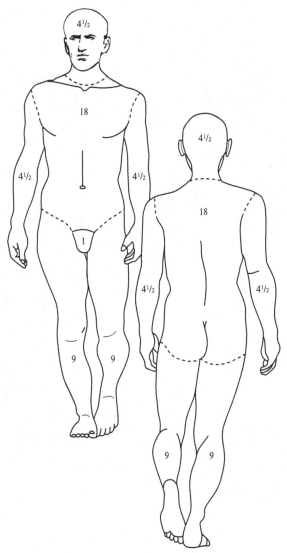

Source: Adapted from Anderson et al. (1998)

Burns assessment area (in %) for a child of 5 years

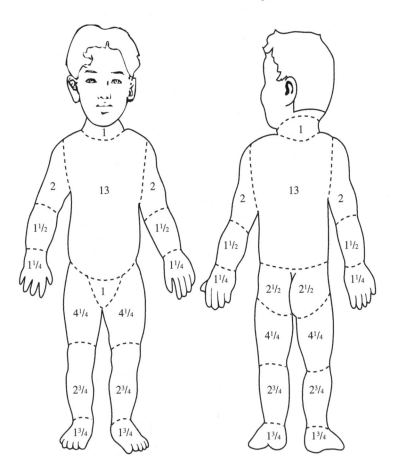

Source: Lund and Browder (1944)

BIBLIOGRAPHY

Anderson, K. N., Anderson, L. E. and Glanze, W. D. (eds) (1998) *Mosby's Medical, Nursing and Allied Health Dictionary* (1998). Fifth edition. Mosby, St Louis.

Beare, P. G. and Myers, J. L. (1998) *Adult Health Nursing*. Mosby, St Louis.

Black, J. M., Hawks, J. H. and Keen, A. M. (2001) *Medical-Surgical Nursing*. W. B. Saunders Company, Sydney.

Black, J. M. and Matassarin-Jacobs, E. (1997) *Medical Surgical Nursing: Clinical Management for Continuity of Care*. Fifth edition. W. B. Saunders Company, Philadelphia.

Boothy, W. M. and Sandiford, R. B. (1921) *Boston Med. Surg. Journal* 185: 337.

Bucher, L. and Melander, S. (1999) *Critical Care Nursing*. W. B. Saunders Company, Sydney.

Burrell, L. O., Gerlach, M. J. M. and Pless, B. S. (1997) *Adult Nursing: Acute and Community Care*. Second edition. Appleton & Lange, Upper Saddle River, New Jersey.

Craven, R. F. and Hirnle, C. J. (2000) *Fundamentals of Nursing: Human Health and Function*. Lippincott, Philadelphia.

Crisp, J. and Taylor, C. (2001) *Potter and Perry's Fundamentals of Nursing*. Mosby, Sydney.

Du Bois, E. F. (1936) *Basal Metabolism in Health and Disease*. Lea and Febiger, Philadelphia.

Ellis, J. R., Nowlis, E. A. and Bentz, P. M. (1996) *Basic Nursing Skills*. Lippincott, Philadelphia.

Galbraith, S. M., Bullock, S. and Manias, E. (2001) *Fundamentals of Pharmacology*. Third edition. Addison-Wesley, Sydney.

Lewis, S. M., Heitkemper, M. M. and Dirksen, S. R. (2001) *Medical-Surgical Nursing: Assessment and Management of Clinical Problems*. Fifth edition. Mosby, St Louis.

Linderman, C. A. and McAthie, M. (1999) *Fundamentals of Contemporary Nursing Practice*. W. B. Saunders Company, Sydney.

Lund, C. C. and Browder, N. C. (1944) *Surgery, Gynecology and Obstetrics* 74: 352.

Mahan, L. K. and Escott-Stump, S. (2000) *Food, Nutrition and Diet Therapy*. W. B. Saunders Company, Sydney.

MIMS Annual (2001) Australian Edition. Vivendi Universal Publishing Company, Singapore.

Thelan, L. A., Lough, M. E., Urden, L. D. and Stacy, K. M. (1998) *Care Nursing: Diagnosis and Management.* Mosby, Sydney.

Wong, D. L. (1999) *Waley and Wong's Nursing Care of Infants and Children.* Mosby, Sydney.

Printed in the United States
by Baker & Taylor Publisher Services